The NHS

Our Sick Sacred Cow

Causes & Cures

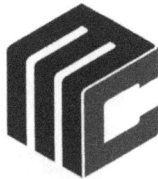

MediCause

Dr. David Dighton

NHS:OUR SICK SACRED COW

auses and Cures

Dr. David H. Dighton

First Published 2023

Copyright © David Henry Dighton

Published in the UK by MediCause, 115 High Rd., Loughton, Essex. UK. IG10 4JA

www.daviddighton.com

British Library Cataloguing in Publication Data

A CIP catalogue record for this title is available from the British Library.

ISBN: 9781399960274

Acknowledgements

My grateful thanks to Dr. Tom Rock and Dr. Roderick Storring for inspiring me to write this book, and to Nigel Nodolsky and Andrew Casey for their helpful comments.

I am very grateful to Tahlia Newland of AIA Publishing for directing the progress of this book, Jack Blenkinsopp (JWB Editing) for his editing, Barabara Scott (Pentalpha Publishing) for her proofreading, and Rose Newland (AIA Publishing) for her text and cover design.

About the Author

Dr. David H. Dighton qualified with MB BS (London) degrees in 1966 from the London Hospital Medical College. After junior jobs at Whipp's Cross Hospital in East London that included A&E and anaesthetics, he became a GP for a short time. In 1970, he took a British Heart Foundation fellowship in cardiology at St. George's Hospital Hyde Park Corner, London, under Dr. Aubrey Leatham and Dr. Alan Harris. There he wrote several papers on the autonomic control of the heart rate in bradycardias.

He became an MRCP(UK) and in 1973 a lecturer (London University) in medicine and cardiology at Charing Cross Hospital, London. In 1980 he became Chef de Clinique (Assistant Professor) at the Vrije University Hospital in Amsterdam.

From 1982 he worked as a cardiologist and general physician in his own private practice established in Loughton, Essex. In 2000 he established a diagnostic cardiac centre specialising in the early detection of heart and artery disease.

He retired in 2020 after successfully making adversaries of

the CQC, GMC and PSA. He now writes, composes music, paints in oils, and attempts to play the piano and guitar. He constantly tries to improve his foreign language skills.

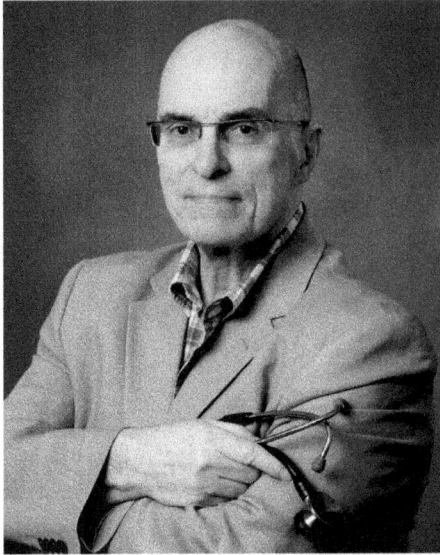

Other Books by the Same Author:

Eat to Your Heart's Content. The diet and lifestyle for a healthy heart.(2003). HeartShield Ltd. ISBN: 0-9551072-0-2

HeartSense. How to look after your heart.(2006). HeartShield Ltd.. ISBN 0-9551072-1-0

The Doctor's Apprentice. The Art and Science of Medical Practice. In preparation.

Essential Ault cardiology. Tips and Tricks.

For more information go to: www.daviddighton.com
email: david@daviddighton.com

Contents

Introduction

I formed the Loughton Clinic (private medical centre) in 1973. From then until 2014 I sat in my consulting room as a general physician and cardiologist, unhindered by National Health Service (NHS) or government bureaucracy. My first encounter with them came in 2014, when the Care Quality Commission (CQC) first asked me to attend an interview. After 41 years of practice without a single complaint from any patient my suitability as a director of a medical practice needed to be assessed. They asked me how I intended to achieve NHS standards. I offered them a case study as an example of what all NHS patients should expect.

An NHS patient attended his general practitioner (GP) with shortness of breath and chest pain while walking. His GP diagnosed angina, but one month passed before the patient saw an NHS cardiologist. When the patient saw the cardiologist a stress electrocardiogram (ECG) was organised. One month later the cardiologist received the result and further advised the patient. Because the result was abnormal, he suggested a coronary angiogram. An appointment was made for six weeks later. The angiogram showed extensive coronary disease, and the cardiologist advised coronary bypass surgery. The patient had to wait two to three months for this to happen. The members of the CQC interview panel agreed that the patient's progress through the NHS system had been reasonable and typical.

I then told the CQC panel how I would handle the same patient in my practice. After learning he had both chest pain and shortness of breath, I would do an exercise test on the same day. If found abnormal, I would perform a coronary angiogram within two to three days. A cardiac surgeon would review his angiogram on the same day and an agreement made to operate (coronary artery bypass graft) sometime soon, possibly within one week. 'Does that answer your question?' I asked.

Why are many NHS patients being short-changed? Why do many die on waiting lists? Why is it becoming difficult to see a GP? Why must urgent patients wait outside Accident and Emergency (A&E) in ambulances, while some patients are treated in hospital corridors? There are many factors involved. I wondered what they might be, given my experience of handling 20,000 private patients over many decades.

———————

For many decades in the UK, the NHS has enjoyed sacred cow status, while private medical practice, until recently, has been seen as a pariah. From its inception in 1948, the NHS adopted a different culture from the traditional private practice it mostly replaced. Functioning in parallel, both have brought great benefits to those who use them, even though they serve a different demographic and use different styles. Differences in efficiency and patient personalisation have resulted.

The sacred cow is now sick and, like all sick animals, can suffer if denied therapeutic intervention. First, diagnoses need to be made which explain all of its pathological features. Once correctly diagnosed it will need sound clinical advice from experienced doctors and nurses. Only they can be trusted to provide a treatment plan that will restore services to patients as once intended.

Since they declared COVID-19 a pandemic in 2020, politicians thought it more important to preserve the NHS than the British economy. Many agreed to it as a short-term policy. Few would disagree that the NHS is an element of Britishness, and must be preserved. I spent most of my fifty-four years of professional medical life as a physician and cardiologist in private practice, but I am indebted to the NHS, London University, and the British Heart Foundation for nursing me through my formative years.

Unfortunately, medical practice as a whole has suffered in the UK. All medical professionals have had to tolerate ill-informed bureaucratic interference, the effects of which have included the undervaluation of the medical profession and the demoralisation of its staff.

Corporate medical bureaucracy long ago decided to control the medical profession by demeaning its sovereign status in society, and sidelining its sacrosanct role in caring for patients. Without change, the grave clinical consequences experienced by many patients will continue and worsen. Once upon a time, doctors and nurses directed bureaucrats to provide what they needed to care for patients. Over the last two to three decades, this has reversed, and medical practice and services to patients are no longer controlled by those who know most about it.

In the UK private practice serves far fewer patients than the NHS. In the private sector there are, however, no waiting lists, no bed-blocks, few juniors in charge of patients, and facilities in hospitals are designed to combine high tech with the comforts of hotels. These conspire to produce fewer complications, a quicker return to health, and a better morbidity and mortality than the NHS can ever expect to offer, dealing as it does with all-comers on a limited budget. This cannot be expected to change much for one fundamental reason: morbidity and mortality are inextricably linked to wealth and poverty, and no government is going to alter these anytime soon.

The NHS faces a serious staffing crisis. Apart from underfunding and pay, one fundamental cause is how the government, through its various agencies - the Department of Health, NHS England, clinical commissioning groups (CCGs), General Medical Council (GMC), Professional Standards Authority (PSA), and CQC controls doctors and nurses. By running the NHS as a corporation (the biggest employer in the world), clinical staff have had to embrace a corporate ethos. While they are concentrating on administration, data gathering, defensive note taking, checkbox completing routines, appraisal, validation, and undertaking audits for everything, patients sometimes take second place.

A medical corporation can demean its operatives by ignoring their experience and opinions, and seconding them to officials with no first-hand knowledge of clinical work. Many anonymous medical bureaucrats now control UK medical practice from a growing number of corporate pyramids.

Doctors now spend as much time on administration and

feeding the corporate machine with data as they do caring for patients. To run the NHS like a baked bean factory, where standardisation, strict protocols, audits, and outcomes are all necessary for tight control, is clearly unintelligent and ill-informed. Where are indicators of NHS administrative success to be found? Is one the need for doctors and nurses to work voluntarily because the system would be overloaded otherwise? Is doctor-exit (Drexit) from the UK an indicator, and are the delays in surgical intervention and cancer treatment measures of success? Are non-joined-up social care arrangements (to offload the chronically ill from acute hospitals), long waiting times in A&E, queues of ambulances outside hospitals, and the need to treat patients in corridors valid indicators of administrative competence? Or is a more appropriate measure to be found in the increasing number of patients who complain about reducing GP availability (some doctors with deteriorating mental health, many of whom feel overworked and are disenchanted)? If these are valid measures of NHS corporate management effectiveness, then the NHS is failing and its prognosis is fast deteriorating.

Bureaucrats will never achieve one of their corporate objectives to standardise medical practice. They may not have noticed, but every doctor, nurse and patient is different. In contrast to the work of most corporations, the business of medical practice is inherently unpredictable, risky, and impossible to control with immutable rules and regulations. Corporate operatives must, therefore, accept a measure of defeat from the start, whatever plans their anonymous, highly paid executives make in their detached ivory towers.

As with the plans for every battle, much changes after the first encounter. At least the military have commanders who know this because they have experienced combat. Those with law and other non-medical degrees who have trained in business and public service management, who now regulate and manage medical practice in the UK will not easily understand the complex workings of medical practice. They lack the experience and expertise necessary to diagnose the reasons for its dysfunction. That they are the biggest part of the problem conflates the matter. The propinquity bureaucrats have enjoyed with medical staff since 1948 may have advantaged them, but it has not advantaged medical professionals.

Many doctors and nurses live in fear of noncompliance and disciplinary action. When doctors of experience and know-how face disciplinary action, they will face lawyers, lay-people and some doctors with no comparable medical knowledge or experience. A medical directorate should replace the entire regulatory system and play a major role in future NHS management. We must staff it only with senior doctors and nurses with long experience of medical practice in all its forms. This will make medical staff feel more secure and less defensive, given the fear they have of being judged by those with no medical perspective whatsoever. It might help to replace NHS corporate culture with medical culture.

The work of the NHS excels in tertiary centres, in its emergency services, and in its fostering of academic work. Has rightful pride in such achievements blinded them to a key issue? The role of all medical services is to benefit patients, not politicians, bureaucrats or medical staff. The corporate culture and perspective of our nationalised medical service in the UK will need to be radically adjusted if it is to have any chance of providing a service of comparable quality and efficiency to that of the private sector. While these remain unacknowledged, and well beyond every bureaucratic and political horizon, the NHS will remain as it is.

In Part 1, I will consider the current state of the NHS, our sick sacred cow. In Part 2, I have considered how regulators and bureaucrats control medical practice in the UK and how they have brought disenchantment and demoralisation to medical staff. In Part 3, I give my views of what needs to change, based on my many decades in private practice, completely detached from NHS culture.

If NHS patient services are to improve, medical staff must regain their sovereign status and sacrosanct roles. Doctors, nurses, paramedics, and all carers need to be left unhindered to care for patients in ways only they know best. Without a complete cultural change, the NHS will sink deeper into crisis, and from one crisis to another. The need for private enterprise to rescue it (in keeping with many nationalised industries) will become progressively unavoidable.

I have used many medical expressions and acronyms which need explaining. For this I have provided a short glossary.

Chapter 1:
The State of UK Medical Practice

A Doctor's Point of View

UK medical practice functions differently from that found in other countries. I have first considered the state of UK medical practice from the public point of view, and then from a quite different aspect – that of a medical professional. The public knows little about the state of medicine in the UK except that the services of the NHS can vary from exemplary to ineffective. The ineffectiveness has deep cultural roots that need exposure and understanding before contemplating change. To be worthwhile, every change must improve patient morbidity, mortality, or both.

The Corporate Viewpoint

Matthew Syed in his review: *Is the NHS Broken?* ('Dispatches', 28/10/2021, Channel 4 TV), expressed the following conclusions:

- It is almost as if the NHS is more important than patients.
- We consider the NHS to be a superhero. To criticise it has become taboo.
- During the COVID-19 pandemic, saving the NHS seemed more important than saving patients.
- We cannot hope to fix the faults of the NHS if we regard it as a sacred cow beyond criticism.

The Current Medical Playing Field

As villages grow into towns and cities, the need for anonymous control grows, accessibility to key decision makers like politicians and those who head District Councils diminishes, and services become impersonal. The same has applied to the NHS.

When poorly regulated, unresponsive business corporations overtrade, their services quickly fail as demand increases. They get consumed by the equivalent of firefighting, with no time to develop and improve. The NHS is one such organisation. During the COVID-19 pandemic, the first concern of politicians was to protect the NHS from collapse should too many patients overwhelm it. While it remains under-funded and understaffed (by medical personal, not by administrative personnel) it will remain in this fragile functional state.

In the UK, a state controlled nationalised medical service is financed by tax and National Insurance revenues. The Department of Health and Social Care (DHSC) pays for the NHS, which functions as a corporation, even though there is no 'Inc.' or 'Corp.' attached to its title. Bureaucrats trained in corporate affairs, business, and law, with a few token doctors in executive advisory positions, control the NHS. Former Under-Secretary of State at the Department of Health, surgeon Lord Ara Darzi, must have quickly realised that his role was but a token one.

Managing the NHS is a massive business operation, but does it require thousands more executives and managers than Amazon, PayPal, or Coca-Cola? No business I would invest in would employ so many. The NHS business management model is too costly, with little chance of improving in the future. Nurses and doctors now undertake a lot of the day-to-day NHS administrative work, but this goes unrecognised and unpaid for. This highlights the current state of NHS affairs.

How expensive is running the NHS pyramid (the sums quoted vary between sources)? The King's Fund (2018) revealed that the Treasury gave the DHSC £130.3 billion. They kept £5.9 billion for building, equipment, and medicines, etc., and spent £11.7 billion on expenses and staff. They then handed the rest - £112.7 billion to NHS England. NHS England and Public Health England spent £57.4 million on 6500 of their staff each year. NHS England gave £28.2 billion to planners, some providers, and commissioners, and gave £84.5 billion to Clinical Commissioning Groups (there are over 200 of them), to provide the public with necessary medical services (hospitals and GPs), but not always in a way most needed by the public.

In 2017, we spent £2989 per head of population on health provisions in the UK. The same figure for France was £3737, for Holland £3907, for Sweden £3990, and for Germany £4432. Jennifer Dixon, Chief Executive of the Heath Foundation, said 'you get what you pay for!' *(Dispatches, 28/10/2021, Channel 4 TV)*. Subscribing to private health insurance is often much cheaper, except for the aged.

How is our money spent on diagnostic imaging? France has twice as many CT scanners as the UK; Germany has four times more. France has twice as many MRI scanners, and Germany five times more per head of population than the UK. The Royal College of Radiologists (2021) Workforce Census said we are short of 1453 radiologists and will be short of 2707 by 2026.

Medical staffing is a major issue. We have 3.0 doctors per 1000 UK citizens. In Norway it is 5.0, in Austria 5.4. In Germany it is 4.5, and 3.4 in France. The Health Foundation, The King's Fund, and Nuffield Trust agreed that the UK would be short of 7000 GPs in five years *(Pulse, 21 March 2019; Dispatches 18/10/2021 Malcolm Syed, Channel 4 TV)*.

A report from the cross-party Commons Health and Social Care Select Committee (2022) suggested an NHS staffing crisis. NHS Digital figures (May 2021) reported that the service had vacancies for 38,972 nurses and 8016 doctors. The real figures, according to the Nuffield Trust, could be higher (50,000 nurses and 12,000 doctors).

In the October Budget of 2021, the Chancellor of the Exchequer, Rishi Sunak, promised forty new hospitals, with seventy hospitals upgraded. Also promised were one hundred new diagnostic centres (at last), 50,000 more nurses (40,000 vacancies are being advertised at present), while making fifty million more primary care appointments available. The health budget is to be increased from £133 billion to £177 billion per annum.

In the Netherlands, diagnostic hubs and co-ordination centres have long helped reduce A&E presentations to one quarter of those seen in the UK. With conditions of work in the NHS as they are, will extra money stop demoralised doctors and nurses resigning and encourage students to apply for NHS medical careers?

Two of the seven NHS England's Improvement Board nonexecutive directors are medical doctors; two of the executive directors have a medical background. For NHS England, surgeon Lord Darzi was the only medically trained one of six nonexecutive directors, while Professor S. Powis (nephrologist) is the only one of seven executive directors who is medically qualified.

The GMC, a charity, costs £114.5 million to run annually. They employ 1236 staff, with eight executives earning between £175,000 and £250,000 per annum. The GMC derives its income from doctors' registration fees, revalidation, language and PLAB tests (Professional and Linguistic Assessments Board). UK doctors pay to be regulated!

The CQC, which is also partly paid for by the medical practices it inspects, spent £13.6 million on staff in 2018.

There are many private hospital facilities UK doctors can escape to if they choose to leave the NHS. Their doors will slowly close, however, as the NHS commissions more of them to take NHS patients. The NHS will thereafter control their patient supply and be able to negotiate lower fees. Are my patients correct when they suggest the NHS is being slowly privatised? The number of private GPs now starting up, and the use of private hospitals by the NHS, has strengthened their opinion.

Private hospital facilities have specialist outpatient

departments, for which private patients must either pay themselves, or seek a refund from a private medical insurer. These providers must approve payments before any investigation or treatment begins. Some provide their subscribers with a list of preferred physicians and surgeons (those with whom they have agreed lower fees), from which patients are usually obliged to choose. Insurers do not usually reimburse patients for pre-existing conditions, drug treatments, or screening examinations. Private GPs are a more recent addition to private hospital services; medical insurance companies do not yet refund their fees.

In 2021 there was a 40% increase in patients electing to pay for private surgery. With six million now waiting for an operation (9% of the population), there are simply not enough surgeons and facilities to clear the backlog. NHS England said they were making progress and hope to bring the average waiting time down to one year. (BBC One, TV News. 22/7/2022).

Most doctors, nurses, care workers, and paramedics are happy to care for patients. Few enjoy apologising to patients for delays, form filling for bureaucratic and legal defensive purposes, and recording the feedback details required by every corporation. These time-consuming bureaucratic processes bring dismay to many doctors and nurses, since if not completed, sanctions and more restrictive controls will be introduced. Most corporations share the same management control strategies, which bureaucrats learn about while studying business management.

How Efficient is the NHS?

In November 2019, 421 surgeons completed a Royal College of Surgeons (RCS) survey. 37% said that because they had had to keep patients waiting too long, they had been required to undertake surgery that was a lot more complex; 77% said that they could not operate because of too few beds, and 58% had to cancel operations at the last minute (because of a lack of ITU beds, no operating theatre facilities, too few staff, and an infrastructure that restricted diagnostic facilities and allowed equipment failure).

On 10th December 2020, the Royal College of Surgeons announced that 160,000 NHS patients had waited over one year for treatment; a fact only partly explained by the COVID-19 pandemic.

The NHS costs £130 billion per annum and employs 1.4 million staff. From 1999 to 2009, administration staff increased by 82% from 23,378 to 42,509 (King's Fund), an increase of between 2.7% to 3.6% of all staff employed. These increases have not resulted in improved patient satisfaction.

Cancer mortality per million in the UK was recently 216. In Holland this is 206, in France 197, in Germany 192, in Spain 181, and in Sweden 173. These figures do not support the idea that the UK offers 'world-beating' cancer management. Source: The Health Foundation.

A decade ago, Professor Chris Ham, a health policy academic, said, 'Doing more of the same is no longer an option. The NHS will have to do things differently by embracing innovation and becoming much more efficient in how it uses the £130 billion it spends each year.' He believes in integrated care within the NHS. What other type of care is acceptable? Is this an example of management executives finally working out that circular wheels allow smoother travel than square ones? From my perspective of providing personalised private medicine in my practice for over four decades, I can testify that only efficient, 'integrated care', achieves patient satisfaction. Its absence from the NHS helped me accumulate 20,000 private patients, some of whom were refugees from the NHS.

The NHS has a new ten-year strategy. The plan is to make many more services online. They call it 'Digital First'. What impact will anonymity have on patient satisfaction and NHS expenditure, I wonder?

What patients think about the NHS

According to The King's Fund, in its analysis of the 2021 British Social Attitudes survey, 'Public satisfaction with the NHS has fallen to its lowest level since 1997'. I have taken the following directly from their report:

> *'The survey carried out by the National Centre for Social Research (NatCen) in September and October 2021 is seen as a gold standard measure of public attitudes. It finds that public satisfaction with how the health service runs has fallen sharply to thirty-six per cent — an unprecedented drop of seventeen percentage points from 2020 and the lowest level of satisfaction recorded since 1997. Record falls in satisfaction were also seen across all individual NHS services, including GP and*

hospital services.'

'The latest survey was carried out between 16 September and 31 October 2021 and asked a nationally representative sample of 3,112 people about their satisfaction with the NHS overall, and 1,039 people about their satisfaction with specific NHS and social care services as well as their views on NHS funding and principles.'

GPs, A&E staff, and inpatients were surveyed with a question. 'All in all, how satisfied or dissatisfied would you say you are with the way in which the National Health Service runs nowadays?'

The resulting answers were as follows: Of those working in GP services, 42% were very or quite dissatisfied, while 38% were very or quite satisfied. For A&E staff, 39% were very or quite satisfied, and 29% were very or quite dissatisfied. For inpatients, 41% were very or quite satisfied and 11% were very or quite dissatisfied.

The King's Fund is an independent charity working to improve health and care in England.

(For the full report, see: The King's Fund and the Nuffield Trust website. Survey first published on 30 March 2022).

David Dighton

A Patient's Lot

Most patients in the UK don't really care how they get better, as long as their medical services are painless, free, and readily available. If only personalised medicine produces the best results, both mutual respect and patients being treated as individuals will be essential. Not all NHS patients have experienced these. With the gradual introduction of medical AI, the number will diminish. With many more patients asked to assess themselves and make medical judgements using NHS website information, that number will further diminish.

Patients seek private care in order to access medical care that is more personal (used as a technical term, 'personalised medicine' now refers to knowing each patient's personal genome). Some are desperate refugees from the NHS, who simply cannot get the service they want for free. UK private medicine can claim efficiency on several fronts, aided by having fewer patients and fewer urgent demands than the NHS. In the private UK sector, as a result, there are very few delayed appointments, rapid delivery of investigation results, quick admission to comfortable hospitals with single rooms, and prompt action by senior doctors.

I, along with something like five million other people, insure to enable me to go into hospital on the day I want, at the time I want, and with a doctor I want. For me, that is absolutely vital. I do that along with five million others. Like most people, I pay my dues to the National Health Service; I do not add to the queue . . . I exercise my right as a

free citizen to spend my own money in my own way,
so that I can go in on the day I want, at the time
I want, with the doctor I choose and get out fast.
  —*Mrs. Margaret Thatcher, The Health*
Foundation. January 1988.

Collectively and unwittingly, NHS patients have become political pawns. Not all realise that politicians and medical bureaucrats dictate the constraints and content of the medical services the NHS offers. When they choose to complain, do patients realise just how powerless doctors and nurses have become when trying to meet their medical needs and expectations? This will shock some, but not those who already deal with bureaucrats in other fields of work, such as building, accountancy, and the law. They are fully aware of the unnecessary extra work bureaucrats create, and how much they cost the nation.

Divide and Rule

'Divide et impera' has been attributed to Phillip
II of Macedon. Julius Caesar, Niccoló Machiavelli
(Book VI of 'The Art of War', 1521), and Napoleon
made use of the principle.

Patients should know that one aim of medical bureaucracy, to divide and rule the medical profession, has done nothing to improve morale, *esprit de corps*, the provision of medical services, or patient doctor relationships. What it may have done is to ensure that students now accepted into medical school are predisposed to follow rules. Those who might risk using their intelligence, knowledge, experience and (clinical) wisdom to make clinical judgements in the future may now be considered ineligible. Most doctors and nurses quickly learn that it is *de rigueur* to play the game, and respect bureaucratic rules as much as the knowledge and judgement of their peers.

Rules are for the obedience of fools and the guidance of wise men. — Douglas Bader, WWII Fighter Ace.

Corporate officials now distrust doctors and nurses so much, that they need constant reassurance from the repeated appraisals, revalidations, and target achievements we must now undertake. We can trace the distrust back to 1948, and Aneurin Bevan's negative attitude towards the medical profession. Since then, medical bureaucracy has flourished, and tried to gain public trust by promoting the idea that the government cares, while at the same time demoting doctors and nurses. Right from the start they saw the gradual removal of practising doctors from any meaningful involvement in corporate NHS decision-making as a necessary policy. For patients, this has been a pathological process.

Burdensome bureaucratic control has now led to many doctors and nurses leaving the medical profession. Medical bureaucracy is to be applauded. They have successfully diverted public attention from what has been obvious to most doctors and nurses for some time - that the public needs protection from bureaucracy. The public should question the proposition that patients need protection from doctors and nurses, and whether legions of medical bureaucrats are required to do it. With statutory powers given to those without a medical education, what further forms of control can the medical profession look forward to? Blaming doctors and nurses for NHS failures, perhaps? My guess is that they are ready to introduce even more stringent corporate processes, designed to improve their control over medical practice. Those responsible for NHS failures must be disciplined.

> *As bureaucracies accumulate power they become immune to their own mistakes. Instead of changing their stories to fit reality, they can change reality to fit their stories. In the end external reality matches their bureaucratic fantasies, but only because they forced reality to do so.*
> — *Yuval Noah Harari. Homo Deus, 2015. Random House.*

The COVID-19 pandemic exposed some of the ineptitude of governmental medical decision-making. The NHS bureaucrats' first concern was to prevent the NHS being overwhelmed (as predicted by an Imperial College computer model that assumed no implementation of safeguards).

What was on their minds? Were they worried the public would discover that the NHS is mismanaged, underfunded and understaffed? They were not so worried that their decisions would ruin the UK economy. The capitalist world runs on business profit, and the hope of more profit in the future. Business often struggles to survive the advice of politicians and government advisers, most of whom have too little business sense to provide parking spaces outside shops.

During the COVID-19 pandemic, the UK public was not initially made aware of one salient fact: before COVID, approximately 50,000 people died every month in the UK (1660 per day, on average). The statistic we needed was the number of excess deaths caused by the addition of COVID-19.

The view from November 2020, nine months into the pandemic, was that despite varying lock-downs in several tiers, infections in many areas of the UK continued to rise. Some form of 'track and trace' system was thought to be urgently needed to stem the viral spread. It took too long to implement, although a massive task. Unfortunately, one must never ignore corporate inertia. Built into most large nationalised corporate systems is something more sinister, however: a reluctance to reduce their inertia.

Despite the widely publicised appearance of the Omicron coronavirus variant in South Africa in late November 2021, travellers from that country could still gain entry to the UK. In South Africa, the Omicron variant cases seemed mild, so any political overreaction to its seriousness might have been inappropriate. Some mutations presented a greater danger (more transmissible with more severe pathological consequences), although some might have been beneficial (resulting in immunity without illness). One question at the time was whether a new vaccine should be manufactured. US company Moderna thought so. The problem was that we had long known that coronaviruses predictably mutate constantly. This long-known fact was one reason why nobody ever tried to make a common cold vaccine (the common cold virus is itself a coronavirus).

Medicine as a Machine

To manage the health service corporation, the government and its bureaucrats need to conceive of it as a machine. This allows them to avoid medical knowledge, clinical wisdom, practice experience, or to deal directly with patients. The performance and compliance of every machine is easily controlled anonymously. Because machines have no feeling or cognition, they can focus on efficiency. Bureaucratic machines need not concern themselves with humane issues such as fairness, respect for medical knowledge, experience and considerateness.

Having had their outlook formed by corporate experience, bureaucrats can be presented with a problem when dealing with doctors, nurses, and patients. Doctors and nurses are neither programmable nor predictable. For management purposes, doctors and nurses, when acting as freethinking agents will make their job complex and not easily predictable. Bureaucrats cannot expect to have the same control as they would possess when running a factory full of machines. Factories established on corporate lines can be predictable, productive, efficient, and profitable, and are not at all like medical practice.

For bureaucrats whose aim is to manage health services like a machine, one step comes first: they must try to de-personalise all of its parts. Because de-personalised activity makes complete political, managerial, and financial sense, it will easily attract government funding. What must follow will be to replace much of what doctors do with apps, or employ more compliant doctors. Both will improve bureaucratic control. Because the idea of 'digital first' is politically expedient, and is conveniently accessible to patients, the idea is bound to gain acceptance. That will leave the rich to continue with their medical advantages: personal medical services, delivered by experienced doctors who know them as individuals.

Like Dorothy in *The Wizard of Oz*, medical bureaucracy might eventually find their highly sought-after digital wizard to be a charlatan. Unlike Dorothy, they may come late to the idea that they never needed a wizard in the first place!

The doctor patient relationship that has worked well for millennia might get side-lined, but will never go away. Only the management systems controlling us and our patients change. Unlike Dorothy, who luckily found her way back to Kansas and how things once were, the UK medical profession must accept that it has been imprisoned within an over-controlling corporate system. This is no longer a nightmare for doctors; it is a reality.

I must congratulate medical bureaucrats. They have achieved the original dream of those who designed the NHS. They have successfully withdrawn most of the clinical control doctors once had. They have done more than that. They have convinced many doctors and nurses that there is no point in fighting back. If morale drops further, however, they risk critical changes in the attitudes of medical and nursing staff that would bring the machine to a halt. This would not be a problem for medical bureaucrats, as they can walk away without taking any personal responsibility. That's one benefit of working for a corporation.

I would like to see medical practice rebooted back to a time when the doctor patient relationship was sacrosanct, and the management of patients was free from outside interference. Instead of that, the expansion of medical bureaucracy has proposed a different corporate future. Total corporate compliance and control of every doctor and nurse is their aim, and clinical Utopia their proposed destination. Most doctors and nurses know this to be a fantasy.

Doctors and Nurses as Corporate Beings

A core belief of all corporations, including the NHS, is that a well-led team approach is the only way to improve their business management. Executives and operatives all have frequent meetings to galvanise leadership, improve team cohesion, and aid groupthink. The time medical bureaucrats spend on meetings is no different. This approach has its merits when the processes and end-products conform to a definable standard, but cannot cope with unpredictable, ill-defined entities like patients, their diseases, and outcomes. If the starting premise is misguided, all that follows will be misguided except by chance.

Personal professional development was something I was happy to retire from. Unfortunately, for doctors in the UK, it has crept into every annual appraisal. Many aspects of appraisal require our adherence to corporate management culture. If we do not express a corporate viewpoint using accepted jargon, we risk being judged as unfit to practice. We are expected to construct files loaded with our intentions and to produce contrived, pointless protocols. We must list the postgraduate training and certificated courses we have attended, with lengthy personal feedback and reflection. We must discuss all we have learned and how we intend to improve (a future pay related evaluation). We must produce questionnaire results that claim to measure how much we have satisfied our patients (easily falsified), and to provide specious '360° reports' on how highly selected colleagues have viewed our work.

A corporation has thus imposed an approach on doctors based on an adult child relationship; them (adult, superior), and us (childlike and needing to be controlled and directed towards improvement and growth). It is the ignorant and inexperienced who mostly think that nobody else knows more or is more intelligent (the Dunning Kruger bias). There is currently, therefore, only one intelligent approach for doctors to take: patronise bureaucracy in order to get the required certification.

Every business would be more easily managed without customers. Without patients, those who manage medical services would have much more time for meetings, during which they could expand their corporate aims and protocols, produce more directives, deadlines and targets, and further improve their management skills. They would then need more staff to manage the processes they invent.

While the corporate remodelling gurus are at it, they might think of reintroducing 'one-to-one nursing'. When I was young, this is what State Enrolled Nurses (SENs) delivered. Now that we have nurses with degrees, the focus has shifted from basic patient care (getting hands dirty) to management concerns (arranging and controlling meetings, data collection, staff management, achieving targets and computer-based analysis and feedback). Their degree studies will have taught them all about teamwork, targets, delegation, leadership, skill deployment, audit, feedback, group awareness, and integrating services. Is it possible that some nurses now know more about corporate staff management than they do about bedpans? Which do they think is more important to patients?

How, I wonder, did nurses help patients before 1980, without nursing degrees and far fewer corporate directives? The answer is that they had interpersonal skills. They were in constant contact with their colleagues and their patients, with whom they developed a caring, personal relationship. To every experienced nurse and doctor, these relationships were the *sine qua non* of effective care. None came about because of bureaucracy, legislation, or regulation. Only a fool would try to regulate inter-personal human relationships, but it is surprising how many try.

Reactivation of Florence Nightingale's methods to improve patient focus and care is now a matter of urgency. Astute, effective nurses have always known how to manage the needs of their patients and staff, with no need to formalise it as a degree subject, except to galvanise the corporate ethos. Nurses were effectively caring for the sick, well before any guru advised the need for corporate medical management.

Dare I ask if overall nursing competence has deteriorated through being forced to employ some who are less able and less committed? The NHS is proud to employ large numbers, but what of the quality of service? I have observed myself that one or two able nurses achieve far more than many who are unskilled, ill-trained or unable. The problem is that the able ones cannot work every shift.

In my early days, ward sisters could dismiss incompetent nurses on the spot. Equality and employment issues now mean they have to be tolerated with warnings in place, even if they are dangerous to patients. In the NHS, there are fewer regular staff members working on weekends. Agency staff and those with less experience of the patients may work the night shifts. This significantly adds to patient danger. What makes it worse is that many more seriously ill patients are admitted at these times ('The Weekend Effect', a NIHR-funded study). NHS England has recognised the danger of this.

Many years ago, when I first became a patient myself, I was admitted to the Chelsea and Westminster Hospital with acute pancreatitis. During my admission, I experienced a few management dangers. Night nurses used to first stop my IV drip, then return with a fresh bag of fluid twenty-five minutes later. By this time, the cannula in my arm had clotted. A junior doctor then had to be called in the middle of the night to resite the cannula. On one occasion, a night shift nurse tried to pump the remnants of a bag plus its air-filled delivery tube contents into me, before changing a fluid bag. Fortunately, I was conscious enough at the time to stop her killing me with an air embolism!

Because a nurse had failed to record the tablets I took earlier, I was asked to take another lot. I refused, even after visits from the nurse in charge and a pharmacist. My card was then marked as a noncompliant patient.

I also encountered undoubted intelligence during my admission. The lady who regularly delivered my lunch stopped putting tomatoes in my salad. When I asked why, she informed me that I didn't like tomatoes. 'How can you possibly know that?' I asked. 'You always leave them, so I left them out!' she replied. This was my first hospital encounter with common sense and intelligent application. I complemented her on her sentient service.

Have corporate control measures that include audit, target setting, group feedback, bed occupation, patient throughput, financial efficiency, and team integration, reduced patient morbidity and mortality? I think not, but who will be motivated to provide the evidence? Medical bureaucrats and executives, managers, administrators, committee members, and accountants must remain fully employed, so they have developed some *'spiel'*, but no proof that their highly structured, enormously expensive corporate activities have brought any clinical benefit to patients. It would be better if all their activities were restricted to a vital activity, and one they are capable of. Housekeeping, for instance.

Regardless of bureaucracy, one thing has not changed. The benefits patients experience continues to come from the work of the doctors and nurses who treat them. This will continue, with or without superfluous bureaucracy.

If bureaucrats really wanted to improve patient outcomes, they would have to go back to basics and learn some lessons. One is that doctors and nurses need to spend as much time as necessary to fulfil the clinical needs of their patients. If this was the only bureaucratic target, patient outcomes would improve immediately. Expanding bureaucracy, the bureaucrats' answer to every problem, is not the answer.

David Dighton

Doctor-led or Committee-led Medicine?

The aim of many committees is to be responsible for safe, efficient, and productive management with beneficial outcomes and wise innovation. The history of committee management does not always support the clinical case. The history of medicine reveals that most innovators and creators of clinical progress were individuals not committee members. To their credit, many committees have helped to facilitate scientific progress and enable discovery (as long as they were politically expedient), and have been responsible for many successful commercial companies producing standardised products.

All innovators need vision. The vision to see what others cannot see, and what others refuse to see.

Corporations, including the NHS, naturally prefer the folly of consensus to personal folly. Working for a corporation has its appeal. Committee work allows those good at office politics to gain status and power, with no fear of personal loss or retribution (unless they are shareholders).

The Machiavellian Nature of Corporate Control

The control of corporate employees is easy, using tried and tested historic methods. It is easy to control those who need a job by threatening their job security, future prospects and welfare, tacitly or directly. Both certification and the need for paperwork can be used to delay or disqualify those unwanted by management.

Some corporations will demoralise their employees by showing progressive disregard for their value, their knowledge, and their know-how. They can then demean their status by delegating their work to others (specifically trained, compliance-minded lay-workers). Next, they will introduce obligatory rules and regulations; the more tightly these are imposed, the quicker will troublesome, independent thinkers and dissidents be identified. Using immutable guidelines makes noncompliance easy to detect and enforcement straightforward. This is a key issue because regulatory conflict can arise for doctors each time they interpret guidelines as they are instructed to by the National Institute for Health and Clinical Excellence (NICE). By introducing burdensome protocols, multiple audits, constant feedback, and tiresome data collection, with a few false or unjust allegations used to create resentment, many noncompliant employees will run for the hills, feel overburdened, suffer burn-out, resign, retire or be replaced by those who readily accept bureaucratic control.

Keeping employees in a state of tension and insecurity will test their loyalty, and allow many to gain favour by becoming more productive. When compliance errors surface, highly paid inspectors will be dispatched to catalogue the transgressions. They will thus impress their authority on the transgressors and other employees. After reporting back to their central office, where a faceless hierarchy resides, fixed algorithms will be used to help decide the most expedient and influential punishments; these being ones which help create scapegoats. Because the regulatory rules, regulations and punishments are published, we are meant to think that their transparency connotes fairness.

The noncompliant have no choice but to accept being punished, demoralised, and shamed as an example to others (scapegoating). Those who are compliant will get a pat on the back, get promoted, or be commended. The ages old 'stick and carrot' strategy works. The tacit message of all corporations to their personnel is straightforward: *follow our rules, and we will look after you. Choose not to follow our rules, and we will dispense with you.* Are the NHS, CQC, PSA, and GMC exceptions to this? Are they kinder, and more appreciative of doctors and nurses, knowing how valuable they all are to society? Are they sufficiently respectful of the sovereign power doctors and nurses have over the life and death of patients? Because the bureaucrats who run these organisations learn their management lessons and attitudes from the same sources, it would be foolish to expect differences between them.

Most doctors and nurses in the UK have no alternative but to work for the NHS. They will need to devour, understand, and agree with every clause in their contract and follow each to the letter. Junior doctors on training schemes will be required to change home many times, and suffer the unnecessary prolongation of their courses. Older doctors and nurses, with a waning interest in their jobs, will hang on, play the game, and keep quiet in order to boost their pension. They will have learned to keep their heads well below the bureaucratic parapet.

The bureaucracy-centred NHS culture fails many patients. With patient dissatisfaction mounting, this largest of all corporations in the world has an answer: to introduce stricter controls by employing more managers, business consultants, directors and other bureaucrats. Some doctors are actually brave enough to blame bureaucrats for their clinical inefficiency! They will say to disappointed patients, 'These matters are important, but they are out of my hands, and beyond my control.' As corporate employees, all they can do is blame the politicians, NHS executives, accountants, and managers who create NHS policies. There is no need for such excuses in private practice.

Medical bureaucracy faces many choices, but consider two of their dilemmas:

(1) Cost before care or care before costs?

(2) The preservation of a sacred cow (the NHS), or the preservation of patients?

Unfortunately the history of oppression shows that most of those who find themselves under the jackboot adapt to the jackboot. They will have seen how easily others were crushed. They may later regret they didn't fight back and divert the oppressor's calumny. Our nationalised, UK medical profession is now too weak and self-preservative to act honourably towards either patients or one another. Where were their colleagues and professional associates when Dr. Bawa-Garba, Mr. David Sellu, and Dr. Henrik Beerstecher (Chapter 2) experienced iniquitous injustice? Many, but not all, looked away, hoping to escape notice.

David Dighton

A Medical Professional's Viewpoint

If you employ a bureaucrat to captain your ship, prepare to run aground or sink if he is not a master mariner. Is it appropriate for law and business graduates to hold authority over the work of experienced doctors, nurses, and teachers of medicine, after becoming medical regulators, inspectors and managers?

'Lions led by donkeys?'

In the First World War, British infantry soldiers referred to some their commanders as donkeys. They were not competent to lead their soldiers, the lions. They sat in safety well behind the front lines, repeatedly sending their troops to a certain death from machine gun bullets and barbed wire. Their men resented them but obeyed. If they disobeyed, they would then face a firing squad. Doctors and nurses are not soldiers, and their dissent will not lead to their death, but there are parallels that hold true for doctors and nurses when they disagree with the bureaucrats who command them.

The trained will do what we train them for, following strict rules of engagement. Only the broadly educated will feel capable to use their judgement and decide what is best. Why waste the education we give doctors and expect them to do the jobs of secretaries, nurses, and paramedics?

Many nurses, paramedics, and pharmacists have proven themselves capable of routine medical practice. I have encountered a few exceptional ones who could easily have replaced some consultant physicians, although with a few important caveats in place. They would need training not to miss serious acute conditions like septicaemia, heart attacks, strokes, diabetic crises, epilepsy, pneumonia, and malignant melanoma, and chronic conditions like rheumatoid arthritis, diabetes, ischaemic heart disease, left heart failure, asthma, depression, schizophrenia and some cancers. This is not beyond the most capable.

Much of what UK GPs do to-day hardly requires five years of general medical education. Capable nurses and paramedics, with secretarial help, could handle much of it with special training over a short period. Their transition into medical practice would deplete both GP and nurse numbers. Unfortunately, neither GP nor nurse recruitment is getting easier with the growing levels of dissatisfaction and demoralisation that now exist. The GPs who remain should hold 'consultant' status, taking on only the most challenging cases while secretaries, practice nurses, and paramedics deal with the rest.

Medicine *is* an elitist profession, with doctors possessing more medical knowledge, lifesaving skills, and clinical talent than 95.5% of the UK population. So why waste their time and talent on needless corporate and managerial processes? All doctors need PAs and medical secretaries to transcribe consultations and update computer records. They can do this from the video recordings of consultations, likely soon to be obligatory for medico-legal reasons.

Hanging in the air is the ever-present, $64,000 question: where will the money come from to fund change? Private doctors must find the money to stay in business. NHS doctors need government support to cope with the added bureaucracy they regularly introduce. At least corporate bureaucrats get all the secretarial help they need.

My guess is that most citizens would agree that doctors, nurses, paramedics, and care workers should spend their time caring for patients, and not waste it on corporate managerial processes, especially income generating ones like applying for Quality and Outcomes Framework (QOF) points.

Since the First World War (when the Ministry of Health came into existence), we have spent billions on building bureaucratic pyramids. They now occupy many office towers while they struggle to understand what medical practice is all about.

As the only experts in the field, medical practitioners have self-regulated for millennia. Since 1948, the UK government has paid NHS doctors. This has made it easy for them to engineer our acceptance of their bureaucratic control. It has required us to conform with the lions of the First World War, and obey the directives of some donkeys. Since the need for practiced judgement, education, training, expertise, and experience will escape the average 'donkey', the essentials of effective medical practice could fall by the wayside, be sidelined, ignored, or derogated if the bureaucratic control of UK medical practice continues to thrive and grow much further.

Changing Status

Has the medical profession lost status and power in the eyes of the public? Since the inception of the NHS, has the ruling medical bureaucracy worked to diminish the status and power of the medical profession? There is truth in both, but these contentions need scrutiny. There are too many devils in survey data, and even more in the conclusions drawn from them.

Many nurses and doctors concluded long ago that their opinions were of little consequence to medical bureaucrats. In keeping with a common corporate strategy, medical bureaucracy has gradually removed decision-making power from doctors and nurses in small but significant steps. Removing privileged car-parking spaces for consultants, enforcing shared offices, removing their personal secretaries, and requiring them to give long notice of intended holidays, are four simple ways in which bureaucrats have demeaned the perceived status of medical consultants. Another corporate strategy that helps reduce the status of doctors with less than consultant status is to give them the lesser title of 'junior' or 'trainee'.

Junior doctors who want to achieve consultant status must complete a training scheme. The scheme may last for years, and will often get altered or extended while it is in progress (keeping the NHS consultant wage bill in check). As the scheme progresses, junior doctors will often need to change home regularly. While in post they may be assigned menial tasks that show no respect for their education and skills, which can lead to burnout. They often experience under-staffing and a lack of team work once supported by traditional clinical firms headed by a consultant. They may have to assume the role of dogsbody. It is not surprising that many resign and choose another career path, often outside of medical practice. Many seek medical work abroad which few come to regret.

In order to compensate for this, and despite the WHO recommendation not to recruit from certain countries (a red list that includes Nigeria, Ghana, Nepal and Pakistan), active recruitment of nurses (and doctors) by the NHS continues. (Nursing Standard. 4th October 2022).

Many doctors and nurses are now disenchanted and

demoralised by NHS underfunding, understaffing, and underequipping. This has resulted from government funding short-termism, and together these have had a significant impact on the mental health, attitude, and behaviour of many doctors and nurses.

Defensive Medicine

Doctors and nurses are now required to record all the information and advice they that they have given patients. The information must be correct, after sufficient forethought was given to it by weighing all the risks and benefits of a management plan. Our acceptance of the need to record every detail simply confirms our submission to bureaucratic control and the acceptance of our professional demotion.

The corporate requirement for more and more defensive data to be recorded fosters over-investigation. This diverts us from caring for patients, puts patients at risk, and is an expensive misuse of our skills and facilities.

The mantra 'If it's not written, it didn't happen!' is nonsense, but nonsense we now must take seriously. Only written reports are admissible as evidence. Other reports and comments are 'hearsay'. We are trusted to save lives, but not trusted by bureaucracy to give verbal accounts of anything we say and do. For these reasons, digital recordings of everything we do may soon become a standard requirement. To believe only documented evidence (as required in a court of law), implies that other forms of evidence are unsafe, and that any trust in what doctors and nurses might say is foolish and misplaced. This is but another bureaucratic step that progresses our professional demotion.

I see saving lives as something special, and an important aspect of humanity, something that takes priority over the mindless application of rules and regulations. The GMC and its lawyers will see such a statement as an attempt to prioritise medical practice over the rule of law, and a ploy to escape corporate control.

A Gordian knot now traps us. If we satisfied the needs of patients better, there would be fewer complaints and less need to act as scribes to secure our defence. Again, I pose the rhetorical question: why would any doctor and nurse choose to work for a medical system, so badly run that it generates endless patient complaints? The obvious answer is that there are too few alternatives in the UK.

We should test every feature of bureaucratic compliance for its contribution to patient morbidity and mortality. Only then will we know which are meaningful, and which are meaningless bureaucratic impositions. Without such evidence, can diverting our attention from patient care ever be justified? Acting without scientific evidence is unacceptable. It is our duty to reject any policy that fails to meet the most rigorous standards of scientific justification. We will otherwise deserve the loss of public confidence.

David Dighton

Living with Medical Error

How frequent is medical error? The NHS now faces medical negligence claims for £83 billion, a sum equal to half of the NHS England annual budget. In 2020-2021, the NHS received 12,629 compensation claims (11,678 in 2019-2020). Manchester University NHS Foundation Trust and University Hospitals Birmingham receive approximately four negligence claims each week. (Sources: Matthew Syed. *Dispatches*, Channel 4 TV, 18/10/2021, and The Health Foundation).

Medical errors are inevitable. They will always occur when skilled doctors and nurses work under pressure in high-risk environments, and wherever incompetent people work. Errors can be serendipitous, unavoidable, negligent, reckless (due to gross negligence), or can result from personal stress, overwork fatigue, understaffing, under equipping, and sabotage (as in the case of Shipman). Some errors are predictable. They will occur more frequently when doctors and nurses are demoralised by working in next to impossible conditions, and where low standards have been accepted.

When errors are criminalised, they often have a negative effect. The exposure of errors can be driven underground, with nothing learned for the future. In the UK, the chances are that whistleblowers will be attacked for daring to criticise the NHS. Many have been blacklisted and lost their jobs.

Prof. Alan Merry, Head of the School of Medicine, Auckland, NZ, at the RSM Conference: 'When Things go Wrong' (26th Oct. 2018), said 'no improvement in patient safety results from criminalisation. In New Zealand, we have moved away from it to a reflective learning process. This matches what happens in the airline industry.'

In Sweden, there is a 'no fault compensation' scheme. Doctors are free to admit any fault without the prospect of litigation in court, the organisation admits their part in any error, and compensation for the patient is automatic. Only twenty-five cases went to litigation recently. In the UK, it can take five years of legal proceedings before claims are settled. Compared to the UK, Swedes clearly value the work of doctors differently.

One of the commonest sources of error is assumption. Since we humans are all prone to biases, and prone to fooling ourselves, it is best to get evidence-based verification before making any assumption, especially when it could affect a life. There are those among us, however, who cannot (or will not) decide anything without first getting incontrovertible evidence (*encompassing generalisations*). They have little regard for experience-based verification (*encompassing individual* detail). Although completely defensible in theory, such people may lack practical ability, clinical nous, and enough acquaintance with clinical risk to take action. Their fear of failure can cause dangerous inactivity. They may find it difficult to balance indecisiveness with the risks of cavalier action. The ability to balance clinical risks and to decide on the best course of action is an art. Once they are witness to it, junior doctors and nurses will not be in any doubt about its nature and value.

The constant call for scientific evidence can be a smokescreen, one that aims to obscure personal inertia and initiative, clinical cowardice, incompetence, a lack of nous, and an inability to take risks. It will, however, save face, avoid political embarrassment, and prevent dismissal.

Overt reticence about interpreting COVID-19 evidence was on display during the daily government TV briefings. Academics and nonpractising clinical scientists clearly struggled to make management recommendations based only on the numerical data available. In these situations, clinical common sense rather than data can suffice like the wearing of masks, a sensible piece of advice (established in the UK in the 1918 influenza epidemic) with no obvious downsides (except claustrophobia).

There is a great difference between having public responsibility (often anonymous) and accepting individual clinical responsibility.

Will repeated appraisals and regular revalidation reduce medical errors? The appraisal process stems from the need all corporations have to discipline their employees. Doctors working for the NHS are corporate employees, and must conform (independent doctors in the UK must also comply). The appraisal process will detect those who disagree with corporate directives, audits, and targets, and those who have no allegiance to corporate culture. They seek evidence of learning, feedback from colleagues (and patients), evidence of complaints and compliments, evidence of personal reflection, personal development plans, and probity. The system costs money, is time-consuming and is paid for in the UK, by doctors. Many corporations regard the same process as a legitimate expense, but would not get away with charging their employees for it.

Advisers have formed companies to advise doctors on how to perform successfully when appraised (at a price). If one accepts the need for appraisal (making sure that doctors are up-to-date, setting objectives, working productively, developing an approved career, with pay and professional progress likely to be linked to appraisal in the future), the GMC should pay trained staff to do it, leaving doctors free to do their valuable jobs. The same problem arises when the GMC and their Medical Practitioners Tribunal Service (MPTS) appraise allegations. Who is qualified to assess a doctor's work, other than experienced doctors and their patients? While doctors pay for their appraisals and revalidation in the UK, the GMC benefits. This serves to confirm their corporate management excellence and worthiness to receive government support.

> *The Chief Medical Officer noted in 2006 that 'appraisal may not serve the multiple purposes of detecting unsafe practice, quality assuring good practice, ensuring compliance with contractual duties, improving practice, and facilitating continuing professional development.' (Department of Health. 'Good doctors, safer patients', a report by the Chief Medical Officer, 2006.)*

Once a clinical error has occurred, patients (and their relatives) want their questions answered. They want information. They want to understand what happened. They want to be listened to and understood, not ignored. Not every patient seeks retribution; they may just want to understand how the error occurred. Many want to know that changes will be made to prevent the same error happening again. Patients want to know what we have learned from our mistakes. Patients and their relatives mostly understand that 'bad things can happen', even with the best of intentions. Doctors and nurses need the courage to be honest and open with patients.

David Dighton

Errors and Cultural Difference

Multicultural societies present cultural and ethnic challenges, and nowhere more than in the UK. The way medical work is now conducted in the NHS, there is too little time to deal efficiently with physical disease. The pastoral care GPs once included in the care of their patients has therefore declined, even though considering a patient's social and cultural condition may be vital to optimising their clinical management and prognosis. Some of these issues are now discussed in the light of the differences between NHS and private practice.

Most doctors sanctioned, or removed by the MPTS in 2016 were from non-White backgrounds. Could it be that some failure to appreciate cultural differences played a part in their downfall? Nearly 20% of all NHS workers (1.3 million people) were then from a BAME background, although the UK population census of 2011 showed that 13% belonged to the BAME community. The NHS workforce does not exactly match UK population demography.

Cultural differences matter. Because in UK medical practice there are sizeable ethnic subgroups, many patients will meet doctors and nurses unacquainted with their culture.

Of 81,000 UK doctors surveyed in 2004 (BMJ (2004) 11; 329 (7466) 583-4), 63% were from a White ethnic origin, 23% were Asian, 4% Black, 1% of mixed race, and 7% other.

This contrasts little with the ethnic distribution of the London population (2011, UK Government Census): white ethnic groups 59.8%, Asian 18.5%, Black 13.3%, Mixed 5%, and other 3.4%. The contrasts were much greater in Wales, where 95.6% of the population were White British, 2.3%

were Asian, 0.6% were Black, 1% were mixed, and 0.5% were 'other'.

From the point of view of discussing the clinical relevance of cultural difference at the doctor patient relationship level, it is important to point out that 'White' in the above statistics includes diverse cultural sub-groups such as Irish, Polish, and Gypsy and Travelers, and 'White British'. It is also important to recognise that 'Asian', refers to several distinct cultural sub-groups including Bangladeshi, Chinese, Indian, Pakistani, Thai, and Vietnamese.

The same BMJ paper (BMJ (2004) 11; 329 (7466) 583-4), makes other important distinctions:

> *There are differences in sex, socioeconomic background, disability, religion, and sexual orientation in the different ethnic groups surveyed.*

The politically correct, detached view is to think ethnic differences are irrelevant, since patients are more likely to be concerned with the technical competence of a doctor rather than issues of background. My definition of clinical competence includes having sufficient knowledge of different cultures, with respect for how people from these cultural backgrounds want to be treated. At the bureaucratic level, it would be of concern if those who influence healthcare policy do not respect the diversity of the population.

Are students from ethnic minorities discriminated against when trying to enter medical school? Students from lower socioeconomic backgrounds (which includes many from ethnic minority backgrounds) are massively under-represented at medical schools, and lower academic achievement alone may not to explain this.

David Dighton

Social Challenges

All corporations, including the NHS, need to apply generalised rules to the way they provide services to their clients. This allows them to better control their management systems, but client processing can suffer when individuality becomes an issue. As an aspect of political correctness, individual differences might be acknowledged by a corporation and ignored at the point of service. Culture, race, ethnicity, religion and wealth status are vitally important to many patients. They are key considerations for patient satisfaction. Private patients will repeatedly return to a doctor only if they find their approach acceptable; NHS patients have less choice. These are important social aspects best left for individual medical professionals to consider, but in the NHS do they have enough time and inclination to consider them? In what follows, I will consider the relevance of these issues to medical practice and effective patient handling.

A multicultural society like the UK presents many problems to health workers. An inability to deal with different cultures, through lack of interest, ignorance, or a fear of political incorrectness, can all lead to less acceptable handling of patients. Who would manage a wealthy Caucasian Christian in the same way as a Hindu Dalit? Like a cello and a violin, they may have similar physical components, but require different handling. Detached doctors, whose focus is likely to be the anatomy and pathophysiology of illness, may prefer to ignore cultural differences. That is for ethnologists, they might say, although they must acknowledge the ethnic prevalence of some diseases (sickle cell anaemia, malignant hypertension, etc.).

Without living in Ethiopia, Ireland, Pakistan, or Lithuania, how can one expect to understand their different values and belief systems? For all but simply solved medical conditions, it is useful to learn something of every patient's culture and traditions. Without considering these, one may not get results satisfactory for every patient.

A word of caution. Thinking that you have sensitively dealt with a cultural issue can be delusional. You might think that you have overcome a culture gap, and have achieved complete mutual understanding, only to find later that you were being humoured. Even small cultural differences provide a challenge, even when both parties try their best to accommodate one another.

Our cultural values develop from birth. They do not change without cultural interchange and a desire to develop relationships. Under such circumstances, some will try to accommodate any differences, or deny cultural difference. Only ignorance, and a lack of appreciation for others (an imperious view once common to the British, prior to the 1960s), allowed some native Brits to ignore other cultures altogether. My cultural definition of a 'native Brit' will apply to a diminishing number in the UK: those whose family have all lived in the UK for three or four generations. This at least respects my sixteenth century Huguenot maternal origins, and my paternal forefathers, who in the seventeenth century were among the founding fathers of the USA.

To see another culture for what it is, one would need to be a fly on their wall. It is only possible to achieve a limited appreciation for another culture and its traditions when political correctness is the paramount issue. What they allow you to see may give you a false impression. A full appreciation of cultural differences takes personal involvement, time, and a lot of face-to-face work; one cannot usually access it without sympathetic mutual acceptance.

Having walked through the A&E of Newham General Hospital one evening, I wondered whether ethno-centric hospitals might be welcomed. They would become the medical equivalent of faith schools. I am sure that the patients I saw there that evening would have appreciated an Urdu speaking doctor. The demography supports the case. Only 29% of those living in Newham were from white ethnic origins (2011, National Census data).

Those who think they understand cultural diversity should try a simple experiment. Try to tell a joke to someone from a different culture. Try, as a native Brit, to tell a simple joke to a Russian, Punjabi, or Thai person who speaks adequate English, but has recently arrived from their native land. Be prepared for a specific facial expression: a blank look or one of befuddlement. Further misinterpretation and befuddlement will occur if you try to explain your joke. A joke will only be amusing if it successfully passes every test of cultural value and acceptability. If that fails, it could prove embarrassing to both parties.

Knowledge of language alone is not enough to enable the full understanding and appreciation of another culture. To communicate with others with no misinterpretation requires both linguistic and cultural knowledge. You will need to know which subjects are acceptable and which are taboo. If you do not know how to approach others in the light of their cultural values, at least try to show an interest in learning.

Without cultural understanding, discord can happen whenever two people from different ethnic groups or social strata come together. Wealth and poverty are also important factors influencing both relationships and clinical outcomes. Ignorance of their significance can lead to misunderstanding.

Medical professionals will appreciate this once they have worked in different socioeconomic areas.

Should cultural differences affect the way we manage heart failure? They are irrelevant when making an objective diagnosis or instituting therapeutic changes. Thereafter, however, an acquaintance with the patient's culture can help clinical management and progress. One should never treat any patient as a number, or as a biological entity, detached from their origins. Few people exist in social isolation without friends, family, or a culturally linked community. These considerations affect clinical outcomes, if only because the level of support each patient gets can differ greatly (an important cultural variable).

Language constantly changes, and this change occurs nowhere faster than between generations. In some cultures, older people are not always comfortable speaking to teenagers, and vice versa. One could study the young and excel at understanding the unfamiliar words they use, words they constantly invent or redefine, in some part, to distance themselves from other generations. In 2021, I noticed for the first time that, 'You look sick' can mean to some, 'You look great!', not 'You should see a doctor ASAP!' Don't try too hard to speak the patient's language. It can be taken as patronising, or an attempt to undermine their individuality. Attempt an understanding, but never use mimicry or mockery.

Humans have Palaeolithic emotions, medieval institutions, and God-like powers. — E.O. Wilson.

David Dighton

Our Health Divide

Why are heart disease and cancer less prevalent in the rich than the poor?

Are different associated behaviours, lifestyles and living circumstances over many decades responsible for the health divide seen in most nations?

Few doubt the current relationship between cardiovascular disease prevalence (including cardiac infarction and stroke) and poverty. Both morbidity and mortality change with socio-economic status, age, gender, racial origin (genome), and culture (acquired values, attitudes, and behaviour patterns).

Clare Bambra, in her detailed review of the subject (Health Divides. *Clare Bambra. 2016*), states:

> *'Why some places and people are consistently privileged while others are consistently marginalised is ultimately a political choice, and political choices can thereby be seen as the causes, of the causes of the causes.'*

Since the poor and the wealthy often have their own distinct sets of values, attitudes and beliefs, they represent not only different socioeconomic groups, but sub-cultures. A culture becomes an entity when enough people share an emotional attachment to it, loyalty to those from whom they learned it, and an acceptance of the values, attitudes, outlooks, and aspirations of the entire group. Internal consistency is important for stability, but allowing for the occasional maverick

49

wanting to break free.

A small minority will denounce the establishment into which they were born. For reasons of political persuasion, a few aristocrats would prefer a working-class existence. Some raised in poverty will seek upward mobility, become wealthy, and enter the House of Lords. A few achieve wealth through sport, entertainment, or by winning the lottery. If poverty and wealth represent distinct subcultures, the rich and poor will mostly beget others with much the same outlook and values. Some remain comfortable with their lot, and do not want to escape the place they find themselves in. Others would like to escape but cannot.

In much the same way, religions maintain their strength by handing down their teachings traditions and creed from one generation to the next. This is the whole point of *madrasat, yeshivot,* Christian faith schools, and Sikh schools. Religious cultures and some cults are more stable, better defined, more deeply entrenched, and better adhered to than political parties.

Wealth and its cultural aspects bring with them many health advantages, but what components drive these advantages? Significantly wealthy people have financial security, with more assets than debt. They can afford to maintain their chosen lifestyle. Some need not work. Ultimately nobody controls the wealthy. They can buy their freedom. The poor can exercise far fewer preferences. Because others usually control their freedom, they have limited control over their lives.

Both the rich and poor share a lot. Both are free to make political and nonfinancial decisions. A lack of personal control, feelings of insecurity, loss of status, loss of hope for the future, and reduced contentment can afflict both. Because of differences in living standards, nutrition and general health status, are the rich able to tolerate stress better than the poor?

The rich need never say, 'I have no alternatives. What can I do? I have to take what I am given. I will take what comes.' Many poor people learn to accept these as part of their *status quo.*

Bambra states that *'lifestyle factors such as a poor diet, of which the "social cause" is having a low income,'* are a significant cause of hypertension. Hypertension is strongly inherited. In my experience hypertension exists as much in the wealthy as in other groups. The patient's genome drives it mostly, although salt and alcohol can both modify it (available for all to buy). Although successfully changing our diet can give us a feeling of accomplishment, it is a relatively weak factor in the aetiology of cardiovascular disease. Few other diseases run so obviously in families.

Bambra also states that *'low incomes and low-income neighbourhoods exist because the political and economic system allows them to exist.'* In this way the poor get stuck socially, and feel trapped with few resources. With limited social mobility, they are also stuck in a gene pool, limiting the possibilities for future family diversity. Those who become financially successful move out as soon as they can and soon distance themselves from poverty. If the poor beget the poor, they will also beget the same spectrum of disease prevalence (CVS disease, if not neoplastic disease).

Cultural identity remains a powerful factor in the formation of relationships and procreation. When individuals inherit similar physical, cognitive, and emotional factors they can usually identify one another. As a group they may refer to themselves as 'us'.

Yuval Noah Harari (*Sapiens*, 2011, Chapter 8) maintains that the genetic differences in races and cultures are too small to explain the persistence of social group differences. Does he mean to reject chaos theory, and the butterfly effect, which suggest that small genetic differences over many generations could result in distinctly different tribes?

Harari believes that widely accepted myths about human differences, fortified by legislation and practise, are the reasons for racial and cultural differences. He claims that bias alone maintains social group separation. But is it bias alone that separates slave from slaveowner, Dalit from Brahmin, and male from female?

Small genetic mutations can kill us; other variants can advantage us. The butterfly effect suggests that minor changes could produce other species, as occurred when Homo sapiens split from Homo neanderthalensis. We humans may share 98.8% of our genome with chimps, but what a difference that 1.2% makes! Viewed from street level, there are enough differences in group intelligence, anatomy, creativity, physical capability, behaviour, health, attitude, and personality for every race to define itself as separate and significantly different from others. Despite these observations, there is clearly some mythological content that maintains group difference and separation. Myths and politics may shape attitudes, but they cannot shape the genetic and biological differences that usually identify 'us' as physically and emotionally different from 'them'.

Beneficial genetic differences have allowed some tribes to survive, while others have died in the same environment. Genetic differences, not politics or mythical beliefs, drive evolution, natural group selection and separation.

The herding instinct of every culture serves as a preselection factor for retaining disease prevalence within groups. This effect helps predict the geopolitical and socioeconomic distribution of diseases of some groups. One important implication is that cardiovascular and other diseases are herd specific, and not just related to our environment. The two are, of course, intertwined. Because we can change environments through political action, the prospect of improving health and welfare exists. Unfortunately this is not the case for diseases like atherosclerosis and hypertension, which are strongly inherited. Health and disease are not the same thing.

Are musical acumen, intelligence, and intellect inherited? These attributes are frequently traceable within families. Some even come to be valued as herd or tribal characteristics. The nationalities of great classical composers and that of many Nobel prizes winners supports, but cannot prove this contention. Inheritance can also dictate features like a lack of sporting ability, musical acumen and intellect. Mutation usually explains the rare occurrence of a genius.

Could the poor benefit from mimicking the rich? Those who try would have to smoke less, eat more protein (unaffordable for the poor), improve their financial security, and live in a less crowded environment. They would need more income, more control over their finances and environment, perhaps more self-esteem through recognised achievement, and to undertake certain forms of exercise (not work-related). Prior to the twentieth century, the poor would have exercised physically much more than the rich, yet more often died at a younger age.

When considering a high protein diet, housing, employment, holidays, and freedom from financial stress, the poor have less control and fewer options than the rich. In our capitalist world, all these options relate to financial status. Increased exercise and smoking cessation have an impact, but not one that removes the health gap (heart disease and cancer are five times more common in the poor than in the rich. Even without smoking, these diseases are still three times more common among the poor).

In 2019 the Royal College of Physicians started an advisory group to reduce health inequality. The hope was to equalise the provision of healthcare services (by further bureaucratic expansion), and education. Will that help equalise the morbidity and mortality differences between the rich and poor? As a measure of the size of the problem, Public Health England in 2018 stated that the life expectancy difference across the health divide was nineteen years.

Is there a way to drive health equality? Despite the Utopian idea being seemingly unobtainable, it is a worthy aim for all societies. It would help if we raised the lowest standards of living. From a genetic point of view, the health of all nations in the future will benefit from the broadening of sexual preferences across cultural and socioeconomic boundaries.

Persistent genetic differences between groups have a prehistoric origin. Tribes that are distinct have usually restricted intertribal marriage. Despite this, something more profound must have happened: the mating of one species with another. *Homo neanderthalensis* with *Homo sapiens,* for instance.

A small percentage (1–2%) of Homo neanderthalensis genes persist in many of us today. Over 70% of all known Neanderthal genes can be found distributed among modern populations.

Bambra's conclusion is that

'politics (broadly understood) is the fundamental determinant of our health divides because it shapes the wider social, economic, and physical

environment and the social and spatial distribution of salutogenic and pathogenic factors, both collectively and individually.' Because the persistence of subcultures and tribes is nonpolitical, there must be more to it. To believe that she is correct is to believe a myth that politicians have (or should have) enough control over our lives to reduce the health divide. I wonder how many of us believe that or would want that?

Political change can bring significant benefits to many, but never to all. Can the poor get all the health advantages of the rich through political action? Is it not naïve to think that the rich depend on politicians? The rich can easily escape the will of politicians, and find a place to maintain their advantage, free from their control. It may be unfair, but outside of the unscalable walls of Utopia, that's the way it is, the way it has always been, and the way it is likely to stay.

The reasons for this stable situation are not simply political. Leopards will not lose their spots unless survival favours those without them. The poor and the rich can both procreate (handing on their genes) well before they die (this was not always so in prehistoric times), so the selection of 'fitness to survive' is not operational in modern societies. One evolutionary consequence is profound. Those who would not have once survived unaided, can now live with the support of ethical societies.

What of the middle classes? Are they any better off than those at either end of the socioeconomic spectrum? They will argue about politics, and take a determined position, but will nearly always subjugate themselves obediently to the prevailing political will. They make themselves vulnerable by taking on mortgages, overdrafts, car loans, and private school fees. I do not believe resentment causes heart disease, but any resentment they may have about subjugation will risk progression of their heart disease.

Professor Geoffrey Marmot, in his groundbreaking Whitehall studies, cites the perception of inescapable control as a major cardiovascular risk factor. Many corporate, hierarchical organisations (like the NHS) have perfected the control of vulnerability. While inheritance is the major cause of atherosclerosis and hypertension, could it be that chronic subjugation can stretch and snap the elastic of those who have inherited them (causing medical catastrophe)?

Medical Ethics

Many hospitals now have ethics committees. Doctors will undoubtedly encounter more ethicists if they are trusted less and less to make politically correct clinical decisions. For decades there has been a move to involve ethicists in controversial clinical decision making. This is part of a wider strategy. Ethicists will reduce the personal responsibility of corporate minded clinicians working in teams. They will help bolster collective accountability. There may be safety in numbers, but the agreement of several people cannot guarantee that their decisions are wise or appropriate.

Few corporations trust individual employees. Corporations like committees to bear responsibility. They also prefer to employ management consultants, including ethicists, and other certified experts (being certificated is to be beyond reproach). Experienced, successful doctors, practising the science and art of medicine in private practice have never needed to embrace corporate safeguarding, but might soon have to if it is made a requirement of revalidation.

Ethicists should start their work not on hospital wards or doctors' consulting rooms, but in the offices of medical bureaucrats. There they will find beliefs that have considerable ethical consequences for patients and doctors. Corporate rules take priority, and can supersede individual patient considerations. They will hold political beliefs including that the NHS must be protected, even if its management is failing. Another belief they hold, but may not declare, is that the judgments of nurses and doctors are not to be trusted until proven otherwise. On the wards, ethicists can be of value on the few occasions when an unresolvable management disagreement arises between a patient, the patient's family, guardian, or representative, and the clinical team. An ethicist might helpfully discuss what is 'in the best interests of a patient'.

> *In the recent case of Archie Battersbee (August 2022), it was three High Court judges who finally decided what was in the patient's best interest. Because he was allegedly brain dead, they ordered his life-support machines to be turned off against his family's wishes.*

Ethicists will respect the fact that medicine is a self-sacrificial discipline, but should medical bureaucrats expect doctors and nurses to sacrifice themselves for a corporation, or for patients?

Doctors and nurses were once the only ones responsible for patients. Now, our clinical judgments must pass the scrutiny of an expanding number of government agencies, most of whom believe that the corporations they work for can manage professional medical issues, even without medical expertise or experience. These nonmedical rule-makers and regulators hold statutory power over the medical profession, and have responsibility for something beyond their field of knowledge and experience. Is that ethical? Is that wise, and can it always be in the best interests of patients?

Ethicists should think twice before getting involved with the NHS. They will not last long unless they play the game, toe the corporate line and risk compromising their own ethics.

Timing and Outcome

The larger the organisation, the greater its functional inertia. The NHS, one of the largest corporations worldwide, cannot change quickly enough to save certain lives. The number of patient deaths on UK waiting lists and the number of deaths among those waiting for a bed in A&E have remained unresolved for years.

Dennis Campbell, in *The Guardian* newspaper (December 2019), reported that out of four million attendances in UK A&E departments (between 2016 and 2019), 5449 died while waiting for admission to a hospital bed.

This sad fact represents only 0.136% of deaths. What corporation would spend money trying to achieve a less than 1% improvement? The relatives of 5449 people might have a different view.

In 2019 Royal College of Emergency Medicine president Dr. Katherine Henderson described the findings as 'alarming' and said that they echo what the College has warned for some time: that 'emergency department crowding kills'. She said 'corridor care' is harmful to both patients and staff. Source: Medical and Dental Defence Union of Scotland (MDDUS).

> *Posted to Plymouth after the First World War, T. E. Lawrence (of Arabia) witnessed the fateful crash of an amateur pilot flying his flying boat into the sea. He set out to save the lives of those onboard in a boat that was too slow. When he finally arrived, many were dead. He thereafter determined to design faster boats to cut down the transit time. During the Second World War, when RAF pilots could not help but crash into the sea, the boats he designed made quick work of their recovery. They saved many lives. To him, the necessity for speed was obvious (I call this 'BLOB' BLindingly OBvious).*

Common sense reliably dictates that the quicker help arrives, the better the outcome. Common sense often evades corporate management.

In the late 1960s, my late colleague Dr. Rodney Herbert was one of the first GPs in the UK to see the sense of doctors attending road traffic accidents. Much to his credit, he was one of the first in the UK to have a green flashing light on his car.

The UK ambulance services are excellent, but in some areas may now not turn up to emergencies. With decreasing staff levels and increasing call rates, the system is failing. New staff cannot be trained quickly enough. Why are staff leaving a job that ranks amongst the most fulfilling? An important question is where has their *esprit de corps* gone?

As medical emergencies unfold, a diagnosis made early

enough will help prevent deterioration. To explain what occurs, one could incur Catastrophe Theory, but it is obvious from everyday experience that some clinical changes will accelerate towards a certain point, after which rapid patient deterioration is seen.

If a doctor does not examine his patients repeatedly, he will miss obvious signs of deterioration. Junior doctors in my day often missed patient deterioration, long after it had become obvious to nurses and ward cleaners. It takes experience to realise just how quickly, or slowly, changes can occur. Whether it is heart disease or cancer (the two major disease groups killing the middle-aged in the UK), outcome depends a lot on timing. This is axiomatic to any doctor with a modicum of observational awareness, experience and clinical acumen. The same will not be obvious to those many steps removed from the scenes of action.

Medical staff should examine the inbuilt inertia of their employer. If clinical timing is not their priority, they may need to change jobs!

Action or More Reconnaissance?

In order to change a policy, bureaucrats with no active experience and knowledge of the subject at hand will rightly request evidence. In their positions, I would fear failure. They are not qualified to balance the lives lost from undue tardiness with those saved by immediate action. Those in charge, caught on the horns of dilemmas that arise from a lack of knowledge and experience, can dither and cause unnecessary delays. The involvement of medical bureaucrats is well known to frustrate those who know full well what needs to be done.

Organisations that avoid personal responsibility, like the Army, universities, the NHS, banks, and governments, will all wait for the results of reconnaissance before deciding anything. They can afford to waste time and money, and tolerate inertia. Research and judicial enquiries can be vital to corporate decision makers. The results sometimes exonerate them from a lack of relevant experience, knowledge, and personal knowhow.

Disillusioned and Demoralised?

Many NHS consultants have quit their jobs to work privately, having become discontented with NHS management. Although many have taken disillusion well, the stress has caused some to fall ill. Others have changed profession (see Dr. Caroline Elton's book *Also Human: The Inner Lives of Doctors*). A few dissenting doctors battle on (see Dr. Roderick Storring's book *The Tyranny of a System The NHS.*), but to little avail.

Why should the medical profession continue to tolerate corporate claptrap? Is it a legal requirement to insist on pointless (and sometimes dangerous) targets, feedback, transparency, audit, appraisal, validation, revalidation, certification, and the repeated reinvention of wheels, all supervised and directed by corporate bureaucrats with little or no knowledge of medical practice? There is a reason for it, but that has little to do with improving clinical performance. Information is power, and the more information bureaucrats have, the easier can they control us.

NHS Culture and Private Practice Culture

Despite the latest fashionable trend to assume that we are all equal, societies are developed by the creative few, and constructed by the labours of many. This atavistic division can be traced back to a time, perhaps 40,000 years ago, when some dissident hunter-gatherers became farmers. The farmers saw it as beneficial to stay put and develop land, rather than roam around hoping to find food. The divide required a difference in mentality, one still expressed by those who become pilots, rather than remain passengers, and those who choose to become employers rather than remain employees. Few want to lead and be in command, while the majority prefer to be directed.

Even as the NHS developed its free services, it was predictable that there would be those who wanted to choose their doctor and to pay for a personal service that suited their convenience. Ninety percent of my 20000 private patients were business owners. They chose to be treated in a style that reflected the services they found in five-star hotels and while travelling first-class.

These human differences lie at the root of the cultural divide between the NHS and private medicine, and after 40000 years, this division between people is not about to change. Even if the NHS came to provide a highly efficient, free health service for all, there would still be those who would want to keep a special personal relationship with a doctor of their choice.

As far as doctors are concerned, the disease profiles of both groups are similar. The differences are social and lifestyle related. Those who seek private care tend to smoke less, eat less carbohydrate and animal fat, and readily commit to preventative medicine. They have a lower incidence of cancer and cardiovascular disease. They also have the resources to go wherever and whenever they want for treatment. The health divide continues unabated. The rich continue to have lower levels of morbidity and mortality than the poor. (Bambra, Clare (2016). *Health Divides: Where You Live Can Kill You.* Bristol University Press).

For those who wish to understand the differences between the culture of the NHS and private practice in the UK, there are questions to be answered.

- Do the attitudes of both patients and doctors differ between NHS and private practice?
- Do the differences affect the nature of the doctor patient relationship, and the effectiveness of medical management?
- Do these factors affect patient satisfaction and clinical outcome?

For decades only specialists undertook consultations in the UK's private sector (mostly NHS consultants). Independent specialists and private GPs were once rare, but are now an emerging species. Independent-minded doctors and some private medical companies have recognised the financial potential. Profits are to be made simply by providing services that are more convenient than those of the NHS. Same day appointments, fast delivery of investigation results, and a rapid turnaround of patients are all that is necessary. In private practice, nobody would remain a patient for long if told: 'Sorry, you must wait three months to see a consultant', or, 'Sorry, there are no appointments available this week!'

In private practice, doctors are engaged in an age-old style of practice, one that has been ubiquitous for millennia, and remains throughout the world. Private doctors charge patients, if only to pay their overheads. Any money left over is profit. Unfortunately an obsession with profit can endanger patients.

There are private doctors much more interested in making a profit than they are in practicing medicine. Would they change jobs if medical practice was not financially rewarding? Of course! The danger is that they will try to sell investigations and procedures to patients to boost their profits. They will claim that these are for the sake of completeness and to comply with peer criticism. This is understandable and correct, but sometimes despicable, when patients struggle to pay. This underlies the bad name some private practices deserve. Those who do not practise primarily for profit will get the satisfaction of working at a level of clinical efficiency not found in many NHS services.

In private UK practice, fulfilling relationships with interesting and successful people is often a bonus. One advantage of private practice in the UK is that it fosters adult to adult doctor patient relationships, rather than adult to child ones.

There are many differences between NHS culture and that of private practice. Medical practice as it was before 1948 continues in private practice today. It is NHS corporate culture that is the newcomer. Corporate directives run the NHS, with those responsible for them remaining anonymous and at a safe distance from the action. In private practice, consultants manage cases without a bureaucratic hierarchy directing them. They are free to concentrate on one-to-one clinical relationships with their patients. Some will spurn private practice because they will be required to take sole personal responsibility for patients, and would be expected to be affable, considerate and informative enough to succeed.

In the NHS 'efficient patient throughput' (a bureaucratic concept, not a medical one) is difficult to achieve. Patients must wait their turn unless someone overrides the rules and allows a patient with a more pressing clinical problem to jump the queue. Nationalisation and individual privilege are not happy bedfellows. To get seen, some NHS patients will dial 999, go to A&E, or feign serious illness. Wealthier patients will find their way around any logjams. They will request a private consultation rather than feign syncope, chest pain, or haemorrhage.

Doctors and nurses once controlled the flow of patients, and the operating efficiency of NHS medical practice. That was too simple and efficient to last.

The new cases seen by GPs and in hospitals are different every day, with only a few predictable incidents. This means that bureaucrats, obliged to work with fixed operating rules, cannot hope to cope with the indeterminate and the unpredictable nature of medical practice. Coping with unpredictable, indeterminate occurrences is what fighting armies, fire services, hospitals, and emergency medical departments cope with every day. In all these situations, fixed rules can help the inadequate, but hinder the able. Under these circumstances, bureaucrats can act wisely. They have been known to retreat to a safer place (during the COVID-19 epidemic they all went home, and stayed there). From there, they could still commission tea-bags and enough biscuits to survive their Zoom meetings!

In the NHS fiscal policy may not reflect patient needs simply because politicians, and the many tiers of bureaucrats employed, are too remote or disinterested to appreciate them.

Reducing NHS resources not only diminishes patient services it also de-motivates and demoralises staff.

The NHS and the private sector harbour distinctly different attitudes and values. For decades there has been bad feeling between the two expressed in sanctimony, resentment, and dismissiveness, especially among some NHS staff who have despised the existence of private medicine. Some still think that the independent sector provides inferior care and steals their staff. They believe that patients in private hospitals need to be bailed out by NHS services when things go wrong. Resentment between the two has faded somewhat over the last few decades as private hospitals have developed their acute services and have been commissioned to help the NHS reduce its waiting lists.

I have known some doctors who work in both systems to have double standards. They express these in their attitude to patients, and in their operational standards at work. Some NHS consultants, working privately, will bring their NHS attitudes with them. Many will have to unlearn them before being accepted into a private medical community. The following clinical example illustrates the performance of one doctor who could not adapt. With no juniors to help him, he could not manage the case.

> *I admitted a patient with subacute bowel obstruction to one of the most famous, expensive private hospitals in Central London. I asked an NHS-based consultant surgeon who also worked privately to take over her care. His management contributed to her death.*
>
> *He delayed an operation, rather than operating immediately. I later found out that this was because he had made social arrangements for the weekend.*

No other surgeon was available to take over the case that weekend (as would have happened in the NHS), so he left the patient 'dripped and sucked' in the care of junior doctors, tasked to 'hold the fort'. I transferred her to another surgeon, and four days later he operated. She died one week later from septicaemia.

The surgeon gave no consideration to any metainformation. The patient had delayed coming to see me for months, having been in fear of bowel cancer. When I examined her, she had a large, tender mass in her abdomen. I chose not to convey the diagnostic possibilities to her, given her very nervous state. I did not want to make the mistake of thinking that an obstructing, infected diverticular mass was neoplastic. She was in a state best described as 'frightened to death', the persistence of which denied her sleep, and promoted a reduced resistance to infection (as first observed by Florence Nightingale during the Crimean War). She had become exhausted by fear before coming to surgery. At this stage, an increased risk of infection and thromboembolism reduced her chances of post-operative survival (in 1974, US President Nixon developed a DVT and pulmonary embolism after the stress of Watergate and his resignation of the presidency). Ignoring important metainformation is a common source of error in every field of work.

Are There Rogues Among Us?

Because patients only occasionally experience persons more responsible, dedicated, and trustworthy than doctors and nurses, they are mostly dismayed to find how medical practice is governed and by whom. Patients think that doctors have the final say in their medical management. Few patients will know that corporate medical regulation is not always in their best interests.

Only very occasionally have I encountered a rogue doctor or nurse. The trust patients have in us is open to abuse. Those doctors and nurses who have brought harm to patients should rightfully remain the main concern of our litigious medical regulators.

When I worked as a medical advisor to Brent and Harrow in London (1982), some GPs I met had increased their income by unscrupulous means. Some were lucky to avoid fraud charges (respect for doctors inhibited disciplinary action against them). Their patients were blissfully unaware of anything amiss, and most were happy with the medical services they received.

Patients who suspect a doctor of being a rogue only rarely report their suspicions. After many independent suspicions are reported, and harm to one patient has resulted, a medical bureaucratic undercover operation would be justified. Regulators think it right, however, that independent 'agencies' spy on both the responsible and irresponsible doctors among us. They will admit this under pressure, but are anxious to avoid implicating themselves. Like the KGB, *ÁVH*, *Stasi*, and the *Gestapo*, all of whom claimed a public protective role, all government agencies can justify spying. The ends (they will say) justify the means. Who, I wonder, sanctions their spying, and who will judge the information collected?

Spying operatives will sometimes pose as patients. They will visit doctors, feigning the need for an appointment, just to check on the services offered. They will telephone asking explorative questions and even ask for an opinion. They can easily lure helpful people into giving information without knowing how it will be used. When their primary aim is defamation, as in the case of Dr. Beerstecher (see Chapter 2), it is completely unjustified. None of this is conjecture.

The Current Politics of Compliance

NICE guidelines, produced by panels of experts in specific medical fields, have provided practising doctors with an invaluable clinical resource. For the first thirty-three years of my professional life, I had only reference works and recent journal publications to guide me. Despite the excellence of NICE guidelines, they will not apply to every patient, and not at all times. They all need to be interpreted in the light of individual clinical context (especially when combined pathologies exist).

All interpretation is an art, whether translating one language to another or translating data and situations into the most apt clinical management for a patient. It depends on knowing the facts, and having an understanding and awareness of the context. It involves the use of personal experience and judgement. Talented interpreters in all fields of work combine data assessment, metadata, personal experience, and guidelines to inform their judgements.

A multiplicity of different clinical presentations for each disease will forever undermine attempts to form discrete rules of engagement. Those with little or no knowledge of a particular medical condition and those inept at clinical work will need all the help they can get. They are most likely to need guidelines and processing instructions. Medical regulators, with no clinical acumen are obliged to replace practiced clinical judgement with rules, regulations, and guidelines. To use them in their judgements of doctors, they must classify guidelines and rules as immutable. They can then use them as absolute tests of compliance. Such acts of corporate insolence based on assumption and ignorance, will prevent doctors from using the art of medicine and will restrain the development of personalised medicine.

> *Many people use maps to find their way, and would not attempt to travel without one. Those unused to such reliance, like the Polynesians first encountered by Captain James Cook, could function well without them. There is no reason to jettison maps, even when experienced knowhow and navigation apps. are at hand. However, a map alone will not always inform wise navigation. Metainformation can make a big difference. The presence of traffic jams, the time of day (rush hours, and school exit and entry times), and road conditions can prove crucial to choosing the fastest, if not the shortest route. The shortest is not always the quickest.*
>
> *In clinical medicine the use of fixed maps for guidance without metainformation will similarly restrict clinical wisdom and common sense from being used.*

Because there will always be some who will draw daft, inductive conclusions from their experience, we must always use caution when evaluating experience. We should not allow this caution to devalue experience in principle. Perhaps only those who have witnessed similar cases can safely assess the experience of others.

For many doctors, nurses, lawyers, and accountants, compliance with a book of rules suits their psychology. A rule-based, jobsworth-like disposition probably helped determine their original choice of profession. Most people prefer a clearly drawn path to follow. Some are so in need of direction that all they can do is adhere to guidelines, even when those with experience and ability know them to be inappropriate. By so doing, they will remain safe in the eyes of regulators, even if the patient is not. Nobody can admonish a doctor or nurse who follows prescribed rules and guidelines, however inappropriate.

> *Imagine if the lifeboats on the Titanic had borne the sign 'NOT TO BE USED between midnight and 5.00 am.' With the vessel sinking fast, there would have been those too scared to contravene the rule; they would have sought other means of saving themselves. Unfortunately there were none. The decision not to break the rule (especially on a sinking ship) would have proven fatal. The Titanic sank between 2.00 and 2.30 am.*

Many rule-based doctors derive self-esteem and pride from how well they comply with rules, regulations, and guidelines. Some will even regard their patient's welfare as secondary. Except for fear, I find it difficult to understand why anyone would choose to comply with a set of rules that ignores patient individuality, clinical status, or the prevailing circumstances. Perhaps we have admitted too many highly compliant, fearful medical students to study medicine? Universities were once for highly intelligent freethinkers seeking understanding. I am not sure that is still the case. We have always needed independent thinkers in the medical profession, but in the strict regulatory system we now have, there is no safe place for them. Bureaucrats are obliged to despise freethinking if they are to enforce all the rules set by the corporation. They have been taught to regard freethinking doctors as renegades, loose cannons, or 'reckless' troublemakers.

> *When a scorpion asked a frog to carry him across the river, the frog worried about getting stung. The risk much concerned him. It seemed reasonable enough for the frog to accede; after all, if the scorpion did sting him, they would both drown. The scorpion could not comply. He stung the frog when they were halfway across. 'Why on earth did you do that?' asked the frog. 'Now we are both going to die.' 'Because it's in my nature!' said the scorpion.*

Propagating Knowledge

Peer review and the constant critical exposure of ideas to other professionals are essential if innovation and useful discoveries are to be made and distributed. Genius level ideas gain little from the critique of others; discussion will help those with ideas of lesser significance. Academic discussion has its problems; interpersonal politics can change the game from supportive to dismissive.

How we perceive the reliability of scientific information depends on the journal in which it was published. The prestige of a journal, the current fashion, and current politics all make a difference. The journal in which it appears can advance (Nature, JAMA, Lancet), or diminish its perceived worthiness (The Essex Gossip Quarterly). To get published, it helps if something new and useful is being reported. It also helps if the author is in favour politically and has a media presence, and if the content is newsworthy. If the publication is for sale, popular interest is important. However prestigious the publication, the aims are to expand the readership and bring in revenue. Every publisher needs to make a profit, or at least an income, if being charitable.

Publishing can get vicious and personal. Some medical advances and discoveries can incite infighting, conflict, and a refusal to publish. Both fashionable and shocking theories are eligible for media attention. Publishers will do their best to draw attention to acclaimed authors. This will further advance their position scientifically, financially, and politically. Publishing belongs to the world of money and showbusiness, even if it also has a scientific objective.

> *In the seventeenth century Isaac Newton, in his quest to be the one and only luminary, tried to remove all traces of Robert Hooke's invaluable contribution to the understanding of gravity.*

Vicious disrepute can follow a false publication. In 2014, Haruko Obakata had to withdraw her publication in *Nature* concerning the creation of stem cells from mature cells using a thirty-minute, acid bath treatment process. It was simply not reproducible by any other research team. Her mentor and coauthor Yoshiki Sasai committed suicide, and her university rescinded her doctorate degree. In May 2019 (*Japan Times*), she said, 'When I dream about enjoying the company of people who I'll never see again, it seems unreal. This fills my heart with pain.'

If discovery is your interest, and you desire power and fame, become a lead researcher in a topical field of work, with lots of politically motivated funding available.

For doctors with a vocation, every medical matter outside of their doctor patient relationships has political content.

Whistleblowing Today

For NHS bureaucrats saving face is of prime concern. Whistleblowing NHS doctors who dare to criticise the system (being a sacred cow, and part of the British identity) will not fare well. They risk being treated worse than the transgressors they expose. The success of NHS corporate control means that few doctors will now risk the personal consequences of reporting inadequate services and dangers to patients.

Here are two examples extracted from *The Guardian's* website, written by Patrick Sawer and Laura Donnelly (11th February 2015).

> *Hospital consultant Dr. Raj Mattu said he was 'hounded mercilessly' out of his job after raising concerns about patient safety. He eventually won a landmark legal victory for unfair dismissal in April 2014, following the longest-running, and*

most expensive whistleblowing case in NHS history. It cost the NHS £11 million. They sacked the cardiologist in 2010, after his warning that patients were dying because of cost-cutting practices introduced by Walsgrave Hospital, Coventry.

The case ended with the Francis Inquiry condemning the shocking mistreatment of whistleblowers.

Professor Narinder Kapur, consultant neuropsychologist and head of neuropsychology at Addenbrooke's hospital in Cambridge, was dismissed after voicing concerns about patient safety, and poor standards of care. Cambridge University Hospitals Trust (CUH) said it had dismissed Professor Kapur in 2010, following 'a breakdown in their relationship, generated by his management style and working methods'.

In July 2012 an employment tribunal ruled he had been dismissed unfairly. It added, 'The tribunal condemns unreservedly the way in which the NHS has conducted itself in respect of this allegation.' The tribunal did not order Professor Kapur's reinstatement because they found they had not sacked him for whistleblowing, but because there had been 'an irredeemable breakdown in trust, confidence and communication' between him and managers.

Professor Kapur, who is now a consultant neuropsychologist, and visiting professor of neuropsychology at University College London, said, 'I raised my concerns about staff shortages and the impact on patient care several times to my line managers. I had a duty to do so on behalf of my patients, but I was repeatedly ignored by the hospital's senior management. If that can happen to a professor like myself, with a worldwide reputation in his field, imagine what happens when more junior members of staff try to raise the alarm.'

In 2017 a pharmacist reported my prescribing to the GMC without discussing his concerns with me. The case concerned an addict who I knew was trying to get prescriptions of controlled drugs from both me and her GP. She remained safe under my care for six years. I realised that the lawyer, layperson and GP from Birmingham who comprised the Medical Practitioners Tribunal (MPT) at the GMC had no conception of how I had handled private patients safely for over fifty years (many of whom were high risk cardiac patients). I thought it expedient to resign from the legal action against me and retire. The next day the MPT suspended me from UK practice for one year. After one year The Professional Standards Authority (PSA) thought it reasonable to order the GMC to strike me from the medical register. The GMC disagreed so the PSA took them to the High Court in order to enforce their wish. They did not want me to return to practice after retiring.

Was what happened the consequence of my being dismissive about the judgements of the Medical Practitioners Tribunal Service and the GMC's regulatory processes? Was it the PSA's aim to punish me for my contempt of medical regulators? They claimed the GMC was wrong to allow me to retire voluntarily (aged seventy-seven, and after years of unblemished medical practice). The PSA lawyer involved thought my prescribing was too dangerous, even though none of my patients had ever suffered an adverse result, and no patient had ever complained about my practice. (see Appendices 1 and 2 for more detail).

When you declare yourself dismissive of an establishment authority, you can expect to be scapegoated. Vindictive retribution aided by the long arm of the law can follow, once any colleague or patient reports you. After all, open dissent could spread and lead others to disrespect the authority of the CQC, GMC, and PSA, all of whom try hard to keep their authority, and our sacred cow the NHS alive and well (in the public interest). It is understandable that they would not want to risk the exposure of their inadequacies or the security of their jobs.

Becoming a UK Medical Student

Would I now recommend the UK medical profession to pupils at school? My answer: I would, but not wholeheartedly.

My advice, for now, is to get a UK medical qualification (which are much respected internationally), then think about emigrating. There is one prerequisite: do some research to identify those countries where respect for the primacy and sovereignty of medical knowledge and skill still supersedes the preservation of their nationalised medical authorities. Find a place where there is an unwavering respect for patients, nurses, paramedics, doctors, and the doctor patient relationship. You will then be able to use your knowledge, experience, training and clinical judgement as you think best. If you stay in the UK, as it is at present, you must face the fact that your experience and your clinical judgement will take second place to the management requirements of a corporation.

If you are politically adept, and dependent rather than an independent by nature, or if you are corporate minded, and prepared to keep your thoughts about any service inadequacies to yourself, the NHS will provide you with a career path, interesting work, reasonable pay, and will help you end your professional life with a reasonable pension.

Chapter 2:
The Control of UK Medical Practice

'We are all formed from frailty and error; let us pardon reciprocally each other's folly. That is the first law of nature.' — Voltaire.
'Let us be enraged about injustice, but let us not be destroyed by it.' — Bayard Rustin.
What is tolerance? It is the consequence of humanity. — Voltaire.

I have used broad terms like 'medical bureaucrat' and 'regulator' to cover those employed by medical corporations (including the NHS, CQC, GMC, and PSA), sanctioned by law (the Health and Social Care Act for instance) to examine medical practices and the work of nurses and doctors. Their job is to judge our compliance to sets of rules, made by government and professional committees, such as NICE and those who devise the National Formulary (advice about drugs).

Government organisations have important jobs to do monitoring medical services and upholding patient safety. Unfortunately a frontier now exists between medical practice (about which they can profess no expertise) and legislation. There are multiple problems occurring at this frontier which need some thought.

Medical managers and bureaucrats have now crossed into the territory once occupied only by healthcare professions. Few doctors feel that this has advantaged clinical management. The methods and capabilities of those employed by medical regulatory organisations need scrutiny (they are mostly lawyers making rule-based legal judgements). This is because their judgements affect patient safety and the careers of healthcare workers, often in the absence of medical knowledge, clinical acumen or experience of patient need. The territory on either side of this medical / bureaucratic frontier needs better definition so that patient care and safety can be maximised and unqualified interference is minimised.

Surviving Regulation

At the height of the Second World War, with the Blitz of London in progress, a building inspector came to my family business premises in Bethnal Green, East London. Because they used corrugated iron sheets in the structure, he ordered that timber and brick should replace them. My father suggested he would carry out the work if the inspector paid for the work. His reason was simple: the high risk of being bombed by the Luftwaffe. To his credit, the inspector chose not to enforce the building regulations, and never returned. The corrugated iron structures avoided bomb damage and remained in place until 1973.

In the broadest historical terms, this chapter discusses a political conflict present in all societies: the conflict between the regulators of all professions and trades, and those they regulate. There is now a lot of dissatisfaction between expert practitioners with decades of experience, accumulated knowledge, and practical wisdom, and those empowered to enforce rules of conduct (with no need for comparable expertise or experience). Conflict will remain at the frontier between the two while those who make the rules adopt a narrow, literal outlook, and experienced practitioners have reality to deal with, and life as an indefinite spectrum of activity.

The democratic process leads the conflict. In its name all rule creation is justified by claiming it protects citizens, and is always 'in the public interest'. It allows for ministers of health to be appointed with no medical training, and building inspectors who have never laid a brick. Elected rule-makers may have the statutory right to decide the destination of the democratic ship, but who can be trusted to sail it other than experienced sailors? Who else should we trust to negotiate the storms and the calms, the shallows and the rapids of life, given that they are all intrinsic to our existence?

When rules and regulations are fixed, individuals may not be free to express their humanity or use wise judgement. These are the intrinsic weaknesses of fixed laws, rules, and regulations, although those who regulate the medical profession may see them as strengths. Whenever rules and regulations are in use, tests of tolerance and humanity should be obligatory, although this is not the remit of those given to enforce them. Doctors and nurses whose work is unquestionably humane now suffer the consequences of such intolerance, but are not in a position to change the offending rules and regulations by campaigning. If they do, they risk being demonised as whistleblowers.

My aim is to give some insight into the dangers that medical bureaucrats pose to doctors, patients, and the practice of medicine. Because the job of regulators is made easier by using inflexible, unthinking, prescriptive algorithmic processes, many doctors and nurses fear any engagement with them. This has adversely affected morale.

Part of a bureaucrat's job is to know the age-old methods of getting an edge, for instance by inducing fear. That edge is easily reinforced by insisting on deadlines. I remember when faceless CQC executives gave me twenty-four hours to produce responses to pages of questions, or have my practice closed. After all, public safety might be at risk (although no consequence of risk had occurred in my practice for 47 years). Their lack of clinical acumen and need for self-preservation must have fired their insistence. By escalating their allegations and requests for action, they hope to wrongfoot, and destabilise their prey. The strategy works well for wolfpacks and bureaucrats.

For doctors working in a state-controlled medical profession, Isaiah's declaration that lambs must live with wolves still has currency.

Very few medical bureaucrats have clinical acumen, but there are doctors who aspire to manage their colleagues. As I write, The Faculty of Medical Leadership and Management at the Royal College of Medicine has over 2000 members (a little less than 1% of all fully registered doctors in the UK). How much clinical acumen they will have when combined with bureaucratic aspirations is one question to be answered.

Doctors and nurses who have yet to recognise the ever-increasing need to satisfy medical regulators will doubtless think it a waste of time to read on. They should not, of course, be wasting their time on such matters. Saving lives and relieving suffering is a far more important job. These are two functions most medical bureaucrats pretend to understand.

From the few personal experiences I have had dealing with medical regulators, and their insistence on enforcing corporate processes, I believe I have understated my sardonic views. It would take a voluminous book to describe the whole structure and functioning of the 'State Control of UK Medicine' (I leave you to create the acronym), but only one sheet of A5 paper to describe the benefits I have seen brought to patients during my career.

Bureaucrats are indispensable for housekeeping functions and for the funding of projects like COVID-19 vaccine production and distribution, but this does not qualify them to control medical practice.

Standardising Medical Practice

An ever-expanding army of bureaucrats, few of whom have any pertinent clinical knowledge, now governs the medical profession in the UK. This extends from the Minister for Health down to those who come to inspect our practices, and who insist on our compliance with rules set by law. They will see dissent as an offence, and as a justification for issuing sanctions, one aim of which is to teach doctors and nurses corporate compliance.

There are major faults intrinsic to the corporate

medical regulatory process which risk patient safety and the effective handling of patients by doctors and nurses. One erroneous convenience used by all corporate organisations is standardisation. Regulators judge doctors and nurses using standardised rules and guidelines when no doctor, his practice, or any patient is ever the same as any other. Individuality and its variations are inescapable, biological facts of life, for doctors and patients alike.

To function efficiently, all corporations must insist on standardisation and disallow individuality. Standardisation is the only basis upon which bureaucratic organisations like the CQC, GMC, and NHS can function. They must thus reduce the opinions and judgements of individuals to one of minimal significance. Along with standardised strategies, they must accept some downsides, like atypical patients dying, and patients dying on waiting lists and in ambulances outside A&E. At the same time, they will punish doctors for daring to use their initiative, experience, and personal judgement when responding to individual patient needs.

The corporatisation of medicine in the UK, which started with the creation of the NHS, is now imposed with such vigour that doctors must consider corporate needs before the patient needs. Foremost among these corporate requirements is the total compliance of all employees to corporate objectives, such as conformity, certification, and control through audit and feedback. Once discovered, they will process failures along algorithmic lines. They will know from business management school that flexibility and individuality reduce efficiency and productivity.

The assumption made by politicians and our regulators is that medical bureaucracy, corporatism, credentialism, and certification are all essential if the health of our nation is to be maximised. Our regulators see the rigid application of corporate rules and regulations (a 'guideline' is too loose a concept for their purposes) as necessary instruments for the successful running of the medical machine.

Medical Utopia?

Many of the politically minded, public service workers I have met dream of a Utopian society in which we all have equal opportunities. This idealistic political concept, while of undeniable merit, rests in part on a biological myth: that everyone is equally capable, physically and mentally, and can benefit equally. In fact no two people are the same, and no two people will take up facilities and opportunities equally. Although this partly undermines the Utopian idea, it remains a noble, idealistic concept. Many questions need to be answered. How is the dream of a Utopian society to be achieved, and who will we trust with its governance? Just how restrictive must it become before anarchy sets in?

In his book *Utopia* (1518) Thomas More laid out a clear bureaucratic structure for the control of the population. Along with Thomas More, every present-day bureaucrat must believe that rules and regulations pave the way to Utopia. Freedom of choice and personal judgement based on experience and expertise must be suppressed if Utopia is to be created effortlessly.

In his dystopian novel *Brave New World* (1932), Aldous Huxley wrote about a contrived social experiment. Having removed the population of Cyprus they re-populated the island with genetically engineered alpha beings (intelligent and capable), with no rules or regulations to follow. After a few years most were dead and social chaos reigned. The conclusion: for Utopia to exist, everyone must assume their rightful place, and everyone must comply with disciplinary regulations. Freewill and the use of personal judgement leads to anarchy.

One Utopian idea, the NHS, remains a boon to most UK citizens, but with unforeseen costs. At its inception only a few doctors voiced misgivings about costs and the likelihood of Machiavellian bureaucratic control. Few foresaw what would happen. Over the decades, standardisation has caused doctors to fear individual expression and to lose some of their freedom to practise as they choose. Newly qualified doctors need not know what has been lost. They would need my historical perspective for that. The decision-making role for doctors and nurses in the provision of medical services has largely been removed. Instead tiers of business and legally trained non-medical bureaucrats now direct all medical work.

It is clear from dealing with those who control medicine that further steps are being considered. They would like to interfere directly in the doctor patient (and nurse patient) relationship. They are no longer content with housekeeping and auditing health management systems, checking on stocks of soap, directing the flow of public funds, managing bed occupancy, staffing, patient throughput, and outcome analyses. They now want to regulate clinical management. The authority given to them to control the medical machine has led to the arrogant belief that they can make a better job of patient management than doctors or nurses. In their view, the practice of medicine is far too important (politically) to be left in the hands of the medical profession.

David Dighton

Who Controls UK Medical Practice?

The sovereign duty of a medical professional holds historical equivalence only to the care of souls by religious organisations. That leaves governments to protect their state from others, and citizens from one another. In every Utopian 'nanny state', there will be laws to protect citizens from themselves.

The NHS nationalised most independent medical practices in the UK. Before July 1948, many doctors feared state control, and foresaw two consequences of nationalisation and government involvement. The first was the inevitable proliferation of medical bureaucracy, dedicated to regulating every aspect of medical practice. In this, they have succeeded beyond their wildest expectations. The second is to make the public feel protected from those who save their lives. This project is ongoing.

In times of peace, why would the preservation of life not be our top priority? One reason is that bureaucrats would have to give the practise of medicine social primacy. Instead they do not grant the medical profession the unhindered right to perform life-saving and caring roles; compliance with rafts of fiscal and other regulatory rules, administered by nonmedical bureaucrats, now takes precedence.

Learning from Wolves

From the outset all good survival guides must point out the most obvious and immediate dangers. Imagine you are an apprentice zookeeper who has never been in a cage with a wolf. Naturally, you will want to know about wolves, and how intelligent, controlling, and aggressive they are. You will want to know how best to approach one, if at all. You will want to know about their usual behaviour, and how they usually respond to human contact. You will want to know if you can stroke them, and if they are cunning and looking for opportunities to attack and eat you.

WARNING! If you consider approaching an untamed wolf, the advice of an experienced zookeeper will improve your safety.

It is no exaggeration to state that, like wolves, medical regulators can also wreck lives. Regulators can cause doctors and nurses years of pointless oppressive stress before moving on to their next victim. Doctors and nurses must never assume that regulators are reasonable, evenhanded, and on their side. Wolf packs in the wild, play the same game. It is one of stalk, catch, and devour. The intelligent ones might try to endear themselves before making a meal of their prey. Similarly, our inspectors and regulators will converse with doctors in a kindly fashion before punishing them. Their mission when visiting doctors is always the same. They are there to collect evidence, not to learn or to have a friendly chat. Some doctors might think they are interested in medical academic dialogue, but that is not their remit either. Some will regard any medical explanation offered by a doctor in defence of an allegation as an act of foolishness (revealing her position), given that it might help with their prosecution at a later date.

Based on my personal experience with them on several occasions, I can offer some simple advice for doctors visited by regulators:

- Listen carefully and take notes. They will never come alone, so have your own witness present. Not having your own witness present will imply that you trust them (they will see this as a weakness, and judge you as naïve).
- Resist commenting, even though it would normally be intelligent, professional, reasonable, and trusting to do so.
- Record what they say (ideally recorded with their permission) to your legal representatives (you can do no better than join the Medical Protection Society).
- Never respond to them directly yourself verbally, and especially not in writing (if it records your dissent, they will keep it as evidence). Never respond directly to any allegations, even if you have a law degree. Leave it all to your legal representatives.
- Assume that everything you say or do will provide them with evidence against you.
- Never assume that they are on your side.

Dealing with medical regulators is a legal game for experienced negotiating professionals, not for doctors and nurses. If you recognise them as powerful adversaries posing as friends, you will have the most appropriate outlook. Treat them as friends, and your path will match that of sailors drawn to the Sirens between Aeaea and the rocks of Scylla. You will need all the wisdom of Odysseus to escape their lures.

It will be tough to take and shocking for some to learn,

but the attitude of regulators, inflated by their given legal powers and righteousness, will allow them to ignore your value to society, any good you have done for others in the past, your medical knowledge, your expertise, and your clinical experience. Clearly some of them resent and despise the standing doctors and nurses enjoy in society.

One useful job for medical regulators is to flush out and remove those doctors and nurses who have harmed patients through ignorance, malpractice, and foolhardiness. This is an important role, and one for which they seem fit. The problem is their presumption that all doctors are capable of the same. They can be quick to make you responsible when you are not (Dr. Bawa-Garba, and surgeon Mr. David Sellu, for instance or take punitive action against you if you dare to object to how they treat you (see CQC v Dr. Beerstecher). They are completely content to follow instructions (incurring the Nüremberg defence if necessary) handed down to them by senior, faceless bureaucrats, personally protected, and with nothing to lose while perched on a regulatory pyramid.

A Conflict of Attitudes

All businesses, whether medical or otherwise, need to be managed. Although not a role for medical professionals, it is a common source of conflict. Those with management and accountancy expertise will have attitudes developed during their education. Their job should allow healthcare professionals to focus all their time on patients and their clinical management. The housekeeping and financial management of a medical practice or a hospital is best left to those trained in housekeeping and finance.

Doctors and nurses must be open with the truth when dealing with clinical matters. With very few exceptions, doctors and nurses are honest, benevolent and altruistic, and used to patients believing and trusting them. Managers and regulators are not similar; they get their *frissons* from discovering noncompliance. There will be those who think I am wrong. Among them will be those who have not yet experienced regulatory retribution.

When making an arrest the police make the assumption that the person arrested is guilty until proven otherwise. Although not quite the same (although it can feel like it), a regulator's job is to allege noncompliance and then to amass as much evidence they can for it. Like the police, their job does not involve giving concessions. Having dealt with both, I can tell you that their outlooks are similar. Both are capable of carefully controlled malevolence in the name of serving public interest. They will try not to appear malevolent, but never forget that they have been given the role of wolves in sheep's clothing.

In order to be seen to deliver fair trials, only courts of law will assume the plaintiff's innocence until proven otherwise. For doctors that 'court' will usually be a Medical Practitioners Tribunal (MPTS). Years can pass before you appear while they and your representatives prepare their cases. It can leave doctors in a state of unproven guilt for years. If they consider your actions to be criminal, they will quickly refer you directly to the police. They will then process you as a criminal. Surgeon Mr. David Sellu suffered this.

'When London is no more than a memory, and the

Old Bailey has sunk back into the primeval mud, my country will be remembered for three things. The British breakfast, The Oxford Book of English Verse, and the presumption of innocence. This is the golden thread which runs through the whole history of our common law.'
— Rumpole of the Bailey, 'Rumpole and the golden thread' (1983). Based on John Mortimer's book. Thames Television Ltd.

A Brief History of the Bureaucratic Species

Introducing bureaucracy and regulation had a purpose: the organisation and control of the majority by the few in power. Only the hope of future benefits for the majority sustained their power.

The original purpose of the first bureaucracy (a collection of appointed officials) was to control a community. Small tribes had no need for bureaucrats. They functioned well with a nominal leader.

Introducing the cubit as a measure was a landmark moment. The cubit measured the distance between the elbow and tip of the first finger, and its introduction provided a standardised measure of land and property. The measurement allowed for taxation to be raised. With measurements available, bureaucracies developed rules and measures for their enforcement.

The first written record of any law created to regularise human activities and interactions dates to circa 2100BC. Written on a stylo in Sumerian script, the code of *Ur-Nammu* lists punishments for the same unacceptable human behaviour seen today.

From the fifth to the second centuries BC in China, many disparate warring states in the Qin area amalgamated and ruled by applying sets of strict rules, punishments, and rewards. They trained a new class of person to administer them. The system (the *Han Feizi*), brought consistency to civil matters. Those in power considered families of no relevance and intentionally split them. Farmers doubled as soldiers and swapped roles as times dictated. Farming and the making of canals and Imperial highways kept everyone employed and too busy to cause trouble in peacetime. A strict hierarchy developed. The thoughts of the Emperor were secret. A firm principle of his rule was to keep the lower ranks in the dark. Punishments were harsh, with entire families and districts being executed, even if only a few had dissented. They added one further sinister element of control: it became a serious crime not to report dissidence. Although much has changed over twenty-five centuries, bureaucrats retain control of groups and entire populations.

In the 1960s the rebellious youths of China, Mexico, New York and Paris saw bureaucratic authority as

> *'fundamentally stifling the human spirit of creativity, conviviality, and imagination'. — David Graeber (The Utopia of Rules, Melville House, 2015, p82).*

Is any of this redolent of the NHS control pyramid seen

in the UK today, with the Minister of Health acting as its emperor? Should independent minded, dissident physicians and nurses be silenced if they voice their opinions and threaten control? Some management courses attended by our regulators still teach *Han Fei Tzu*, and you will see evidence of it. Chinese legalism (Fa-Jia) worked well in opposing Confucianism (with its focus on respect for individuals) twenty-five centuries ago, and it works well today, albeit with a little reluctant respect for individuals, paid as a lip-service to the democratic principle.

Over the centuries regulation has softened, and bureaucrats have introduced more subtle means of control. The taxes and mortgages younger people pay function to keep them from troublemaking. The rich are too busy investing their money, spending their money, avoiding tax, and enjoying themselves to bother with dissidence. Some of the super-rich become political party donors and can influence power whenever it is in their interest to do so.

Only those who despise compliance and conformity (now called extremists) present a danger to bureaucracy and regulators. When regulation infringes our liberties too much, the dissident revolt, carrying many compliant people with them. Autocratic regulators know that compliance can quickly turn to instability, especially if facilitated by modern mobile media communication platforms. Regulators know full well that any oppression they mete out has its limits. If doctors are oppressed after writing about CQC inspections (Dr. Beerstecher), and the GMC wrongly dismisses doctors for wrongdoing (Dr. Hadiza Bawa-Garba, and Mr David Sellu), they risk testing the threshold of rebellious discontent. At that threshold, demoralised and disenchanted doctors might consider backlash action, albeit inhibited by worries about their future job security.

Any attempt to 'deregulate' (to change regulatory structure and reduce bureaucracy), results in

> *'a fivefold increase in the actual number of forms to be filled in, reports to be filed, rules and regulations for lawyers to interpret, and an expansion of the numbers of officious people in offices whose entire job seems to be to provide convoluted explanations for why one may not do things'.* — *David Graeber (2015), The Utopia of Rules, p 17.*

Our Medical Regulators

An Act of Parliament formed the Care Quality Commission (CQC) in 2009. The CQC brought health and social care regulation in England under one roof. The CQC merged the operations of the Healthcare Commission, the Commission for Social Care Inspection, and the Mental Health Act Commission.

The year 1858 saw the establishment of the General Council of Medical Education and Registration of the United Kingdom. It is now the General Medical Council (GMC). Their original role was to take charge of registration and medical education across the UK, and to publish a pharmacopoeia listing available drugs and directions for their use.

Before the GMC was established, there were nineteen bodies regulating the UK medical profession. All bodies used different tests to judge clinical competence. Even the Archbishop of Canterbury had a right to issue a license to practice. The 1841 Census estimated that one third of doctors in England were 'unqualified' (uncertificated, but not necessarily incapable of safe medical practice).

The NHS Reform and Health Care Professions Act of 2002 gave rise to the Professional Standards Authority (PSA). The most recent legislation was the Health and Social Care Act (2012), which gave to them responsibilities relating to Accredited Registers. They advise the Privy Council on appointments to the nine regulators' councils. They have authority to:

- Review decisions made by the nine regulators about medical practitioners' 'fitness to practice', and the power to appeal decisions to the High Court (Court of Session in Scotland) if considered insufficient to protect the public.
- Accredit voluntary registers that meet their standards, suspend or remove accreditation, and apply conditions.

You will read later that they thought me too noncompliant and unfit (dangerous) to continue in practice. They did not want the GMC to allow the voluntary resignation of my licence to practice (one year after I retired). They wanted me struck from the register so that my reapplication (which I never intended to complete having retired) would be unlikely to succeed. They took the GMC to the High Court in order to get their way, and won.

David Dighton

Big Simple Things

Governments are good at doing big, simple things. Cave dwellers were capable of something similar when wielding large clubs as weapons. Helping patients meaningfully requires knowledge of medical science, a facility for the art of medicine and tools that are much more refined.

The government assigned 'Tier 3' measures to the City of Liverpool. These were measures to restrict the spread of COVID-19 (put into place on 13/10/2020). Both the numbers infected and the rate of change in the incidence of such infections had been rising. The measures imposed as a result allowed some restaurants to remain open, while bars had to close.

A bar owner interviewed on BBC TV made an important point about blanket bureaucratic measures. 'Why don't they allow those fully compliant businesses with good preventative measures in place to remain open while those who flaunt sensible prophylactic rules (wearing masks, washing hands, and maintaining a safe distance) are closed?'

We allow medical bureaucrats who have no medical or scientific education to bypass clinical detail. If you become a detail, like the bar owner, be prepared to suffer. No patient, doctor, or nurse should have to suffer bureaucratic decisions that lack common sense and any consideration of individuality.

The Body Corporate

In 1948 politicians decided that medical practice was far too important to be left to the medical profession. Creating the NHS embodied the view.

The NHS is a corporation managed on business principles, with medical principles trailing behind. It is run by those with MBAs, legal degrees, and a political orientation rather than medical degrees. Through group consensus meetings, inspection, audit, feedback, and the rigid enforcement of rules and regulations, their desire is to standardise medical activity. Without standardisation there can be no proper control and regulation. Their aim is to control the performance of every health employee.

Corporate standardisation means the rejection of local knowledge, local practice, and common sense, since policy can only be decided at the head office. Important details, like demography can be ignored. To remain in control, their committees will readily forsake wise judgement, individual action, and the best of outcomes.

Megalithic structures and organisations like the NHS all have intrinsic inertia. Their speed of adaption and responses can only be cumbersome and slow. Every megalithic organisation (including those that regulate the medical profession) will find it difficult to employ more than fixed thought and standardised processing. So that it can function at all, every corporate system is forced to adopt crude, unjust strategies when dealing with individuals (doctors, nurses, and patients). They cannot easily cope with variants. By contrast, dealing with human variation is intrinsic to medical practice.

Don't expect to convince any megalith corporation that you or your patients differ from the average and deserve individual consideration. Their size compels them to adhere to immutable rules, fixed assumptions, generalisations, and standards agreed by the controlling board, often with no direct experience of the business. While this will serve the majority who favour the product or service, there will be many not so well served, except by chance. The corporate NHS, purporting to serve all, is bound to dissatisfy many with its limited responsiveness to individual patients and situations, even if free at the point of service. Working at a much smaller scale, private practices and hospitals are not bound by the same inertia.

The work of doctors and nurses could not be more different from those who direct and manage corporations. For all doctors and nurses some procedural standardisation is desirable, but then the uncertainty of patient biological variance provides a challenge: no patient, or his medical condition, is ever exactly the same as another (although many are close enough). We cannot conveniently tie down every clinical intervention to an exactly standardised procedure, although the attempt advantages the inexperienced and those in training.

Inventive, artistic freewill expresses the opposite of standardisation. Doctors who aspire to practise the art of medicine will find themselves in conflict with regulators whose mission is to enforce standard rules and procedures, some of which may be clinically inappropriate. The art of medicine requires each patient to be considered as an individual within the context of their own life.

What do doctors and nurses think about the loss of autonomy corporatisation has brought them? In the company of doctors and nurses, many will remark how disenfranchised they feel in the face of medical bureaucratic control and intervention. Many fear that their name will be flagged up on some medical regulator's radar, and assigned to a database somewhere. In keeping with other law enforcement agencies, those with allegations against them will have their name recorded permanently, even after being found innocent. Regulatory authorities might claim this to be a misconception. If they think it to be 'in the public interest', they will do it as a matter of good corporate governance. All corporations do it to maintain an impression of 'transparency'.

Doctors and nurses know perfectly well that bureaucrats can create inappropriate medical policies and actions. Yet, through fear of them, few will argue and fight back. We are all keen to comment, but few of us make any attempt to bring about change. Those who try know they are likely to be invited to accept Sisyphus' fate.

Our regulators, geared for legal adversarial processes, will base their views on the documented evidence they can understand and choose to accept. They can choose to overlook the clinical context, back-story, and metainformation that may apply to you, and your patients (they will assign it to unreliable opinion and hearsay). Expect no medical academic discussion about the clinical relevance of rules and guidelines. Like most enforcers they have no appetite, ability, or need for reasoned clinical argument. Their job is to rehearse and enforce directives written, as far as they are concerned, on tablets of stone. Some will even adopt a biblical air of authority, with a mission that can seem Messianic.

With regulators having the sole purpose of enforcing standardised rules, they can limit themselves to a binary judgement such as deciding whether or not a doctor or nurse has been compliant. Among the accepted rules are those set out in the GMC's 'Good Medical Practice'. At MPTS tribunals, they will regard these clinical guidelines as fixed rules if it suits them. They will also co-opt NICE guidelines and BNF 'guidance' as if they were immutable, and use them for enforcement. Academic considerations are not for them. In the absence of medical education and clinical nous, this is understandable, but technically outrageous. Why would any experienced clinician adopt a guideline when, in his experienced judgement, it is clinically inappropriate? This alone will make some MPTS decisions unsafe.

A Job too Risky?

Nothing concerns medical bureaucrats more than medical risk taking and the mistakes doctors make. Those who cannot handle risk and are not prepared for mistakes while helping others and saving their lives should never consider the medical profession as a career. It does, however, explain why some doctors choose bureaucracy or academia.

Doctors and nurses work in a high-risk environment with risks that are intrinsic to the job. We cannot expect regulatory officials to appreciate the true life and death risks faced daily by doctors. Doctors do not take one risk occasionally like bureaucrats, they take many every day. Doctors must identify and grade clinical risk, and manage it continuously. Bureaucrats learn to delegate (pass the buck) and let committees decide. They will never have to jeopardise their jobs by taking risks. They are clearly not people to ask about clinical risk, yet we permit them to assess the work of doctors. With no medical experience it is understandable that they regard every clinical risk as frightening and unacceptable.

Without constantly practising risk assessment and reviewing the results it is impossible to function effectively as a doctor. The sovereignty patients afford us implies that they trust us to take life and death decisions on their behalf. Those so trusted at a personal level find themselves in a position matched by no other profession.

> *Give too much diuretic, and a patient in heart failure will experience the effects of reducing systemic perfusion (peripheral blood flow); give too much digoxin and the patient's cardiac function will not improve further without side-effects; give too little anticoagulant and thrombi may form; give too much anticoagulant and they could bleed to death. These everyday examples of balancing therapeutic risk illustrate the art needed to practise medicine. If patients are to be kept safe and benefit, basic knowledge is not enough. All balancing acts need practice. Expertise comes from balancing situations so that risks are kept to a minimum.*

Through clinical experience unavailable to outsiders, doctors learn to manage clinical risk and patient satisfaction. Because chance is always involved, the very nature of clinical risk-taking means that mistakes will occur. Even though mistakes are inevitable, doctors are duty bound to try their best to help each patient, whatever the difficulty, the time limits, and other restraints. We are required to be openminded at all times, to admit our mistakes, and to learn from them. Many mistakes are serendipitous or result from a lack of expertise, rather than through intention or through being callous. Dealing with them humanely will mark our altruism and dedication to

102

patients. Even if medical bureaucrats find it difficult to accept, few patients believe that medical intervention is risk free, and most believe that doctors and nurses try their best to avoid it.

Patients are the first to appreciate our dedication when mistakes occur. What they object to most are mistakes that are not admitted, fully discussed, or apologised for. Patients do not want mistakes to be ignored or repeated. They want others to benefit from their acknowledgement.

When doctors and nurses admit to a mistake, even when done in good faith, they must prepare themselves for what might come next. That could be a posse of case supervisors and *pro bono* lawyers working for the patient, the GMC, the police or the CQC, searching for evidence of guilt. Since none of them will have anything to lose (except their jobs, if they don't get convictions), all nurses and doctors must seek legal representation from the very first moment. Do nothing, say nothing, and write nothing, until you have taken legal advice. My advice is to contact the MPS, and ask to be represented by a competent solicitor. Mr. A. L. of Radcliffe's Le Brasseur, London, was mine, and I could not have done better.

The way medical bureaucrats and regulators handle doctors can be frightening - frightening enough to make some leave the UK medical profession. If we are to put a stop to a further 'Drexit', changes in regulation and bureaucratic activity are necessary. As an interim step before any legislative change can occur, regulators will need to change their orientation and attitude; from one that is punitive and seeks scapegoats ('Fascist', Madeleine Albright calls this) to an attitude that is reasonable, considerate, conciliatory, and understanding.

Legislative change will happen only if the public find out how regulators treat doctors and help us apply political pressure. Regulators will need to be trained to respect us more for the work we do and despise us less for the obvious privileges we enjoy like the respect of patients and the sovereignty they grant us over their life and death.

Our regulators, content with the *status quo* and their high salaries, do not need to support change. All medical regulatory bodies need to regain their former humble public servant status, and the subservient state of mind that was appropriate to their role. They will of course fight vehemently to preserve their current sanctimonious status and their right to practice some insolence of power.

Most doctors and nurses are too scared, too naïve, or too disinterested to get involved in changing regulation. We mostly choose to keep our heads below the parapet and avoid exposure to snipers. While the current level of fear of regulators continues, the medical profession will remain in a 'catch 22' situation, having to tolerate regulators who know nothing about medicine but have an unacceptable level of control over us and medical practice.

Clinical Risk

The absence of a medical education and clinical experience should inhibit regulators and lawyers from assessing clinical risk, but it doesn't. Despite a lack of medical expertise, regulators will punish doctors and nurses for what they see as 'their potential risk to the public, and public safety'. The best they can do is to ask third-party doctors what they think. They too will be limited to the general case, and to abstractions that take no account of a doctor (or a patient) as an individual, or the academic validity of their ideas and methods. They will simply quote published evidence and go no further into matters of personal context. Many do their best with the limited information at their disposal. If they ask for more information, it can be short of metadata. Hopefully, they know that the metainformation can be crucial to safely forming opinions and wise judgement. Still, it's a job. It pays well, and most want to hang on to it.

Regulators are free to speculate on what future harm a doctor or nurse might cause the public, and thus whether they should continue in practice. They will do this even if there is no evidence of previous harm, as in my case (see the description of my case considered by the MPTS in Appendix 1, and by the PSA in Appendix 2). To act in a failsafe manner, they have to guess. They will need to catastrophise about what might befall patients in the future. Since they know that guesswork is unsafe, they will do what seems sensible and adopt failsafe policies. When in any doubt, it is obviously safer for them to sanction a doctor, or remove him rather than let him continue. All policies, failsafe or otherwise, are unsafe when formed by those with no pertinent clinical knowledge and using guesswork.

I doubt they have vengeance in mind, but it is part of their mission to teach doctors reformative lessons. They can achieve this using scapegoats. Before concluding their deliberations and passing sentence, they expect every medical professional who comes before them to express as much heartfelt contrition, remorse, regret, and penitence as possible (which is good for their public image), even when no harm has come to any patient (as in my case). They will use the remorse expressed as a measure of their readiness to comply in the future. Having brought no harm to any of my 20,000 patients in over fifty years of practise, I disagreed with their evaluation of my clinical performance. I thus refused to show them contrition, and had no reason to apologise to my patient (her opinion, and mine).

It will be an unenlightening experience for most practising doctors to deal with any allegation made by medical bureaucrats. Expect to come face to face with their corporate expectations and what they like to project: their fearsome bureaucratic authority. There is nothing to be learned, except to find out how little they know about medical practice and how it pleases them to exercise their authority. After encountering some of them, you might become clearer about the need for bureaucratic reform.

To set the current regulatory scene into perspective, I will now indulge in a little mutinous parody.

Draft Memo to all Medical Bureaucrats

STRICTLY CONFIDENTIAL

From: The Health Ministry Control Centre (2023)
13th Floor, Ivory Towers,
Whitehall St.,
London. UK.
Future Medical Service Provision

Political and economic aims once centred on managing physical survival. They have now progressed beyond this basic requirement. Public services and their convenience are now major public priorities. Our role is to decide what compromises to medical services will keep them satisfied. Because of underfunding, we cannot support much of what doctors and nurses think best for patient centred care.

As bureaucrats in control of the health of our nation, we

strive continually to convince the electorate of our worth, although a few contentious directives made by medical bureaucrats during the COVID-19 pandemic did not promote our public image as we might have wished.(No new PARA) Doctors, nurses, and all health workers, however, gained much kudos throughout the pandemic. The public needs to appreciate that the NHS is safe in our hands and we are here to protect them from the many risks they face from medical professionals.

By demonstrating our knowledge, intelligence, worthiness, usefulness and sincerity, we aim to stop any erosion of public faith in us. We need to show that we are worthy of their trust, and can meet their expectations by providing ready access to all essential public services 24/7. Voters must be able to take certain public services for granted: refuse collection, sewage treatment, a police and fire service, and a health service which, thankfully, they believe to be the best in the world. Voters pay their taxes and demand these services as a right.

Medical operatives (doctors, nurses, and medical ancillary workers) have long regarded their profession as sacrosanct. They feel they have nothing to learn from bureaucrats and politicians (seen to seek power and control over them), or those in business determined to accumulate wealth and personal gratification. Although we acknowledge their altruism, we also recognise it as a weakness. The altruistic among them will rarely strike, whatever we demand from them.

The provision of public medical services is now an expensive but crucially important political issue. For these reasons we must keep control and never pass it to those who claim to know most about it: doctors, nurses, and other healthcare workers. We could, of course, consider passing some control over to them, but only to get them blamed for any failure.

We must keep medical intervention affordable. For this reason, medical service costs will need constant review, so that they comply with the strictest of fiscal and managerial constraints. Doctors will always want the latest, expensive equipment, in order to perform their 'state-of-the-art' techniques. They will argue that this is what all patients deserve, although using such techniques will also gain them personal prestige. This unaffordable, altruistic trait of doctors and nurses is best disregarded. We must counter the freedom doctors seek to do what they think is best for patients with the priorities we set them, even though we cannot claim any equivalent medical expertise. Targets matter and audits must continue to prove value for the money we spend.

In order to save money on senior staff salaries, we must keep junior doctors in training for longer, and make certification harder to get.

Instead of regarding themselves as independent, respected, altruistic professionals dedicated to patient welfare and the improvement of patient health, doctors and nurses should come to see themselves as state managed operatives. We must teach them that the health system is far too important politically for them to control and manage.

To ensure tight political control over health services in the future, we need to influence medical student selection criteria. Any compassionate trait, a desire to help others, or an intention to advance medical science should not get priority over those who express strong compliance to rules by nature, and allegiance to authority. It will help maintain our control if we choose only those who are dispassionate, preferably in need of a job (after imposing university fees, many will remain in our debt), and who show a submissive, compliant nature. They must respect our rules, regulations, and politically expedient directives above any personal or academic considerations. There is an advantage to allowing the entry of foreign doctors. While they work here, their visas are in our gift. This will assure their compliance.

These days there is not much need for clinical experience and academic prowess (academics are mostly dissidents). We can soon replace these with something more reliable: Artificial Intelligence (AI) Systems. They will make large financial savings possible. We will continue to discourage doctors who practise the art of medicine, since it is impossible to measure and regulate. It takes up far too much consulting time and excessively devours valuable human resources. Patients warm to the approach, but it cannot be justified financially. What we need is maximal patient throughput and functional efficiency. Tight financial and managerial controls will remain in place to support these aims.

In time, AI will help reduce the numbers of doctors and nurses. We will need to train more nurse-practitioners, pharmacists, and paramedics to replace them. AI in the hands of nurses, could make many GPs obsolete. Practices could be closed, and yet more money saved. We need to do this slowly to avoid adverse public reaction. The public already tolerate restricted GP availability, and fewer emergency and personal services. Initially it will lose votes, but like all other political changes, the public will simply get used to it, given time. They will quickly adapt. Only the ardent few will bother to resist our fait accompli.

Keeping patients happy and grateful to the NHS is crucial. Reject all attempts to provide individual personal care, or any progression towards a service which aims to provide effective relationships, lengthy consultations, patient continuity, or accurate assessments and diagnosis. Fortunately young patients and doctors know nothing about personal care, and nobody misses what they never had. Older patients and doctors who favour a personalised approach are a diminishing cohort. We can ignore their protests about 'changes for the worse'.

Dismiss whenever you can the use of the latest (ever more expensive) techniques, apparatus, and research. They are all too expensive. World economic conditions are difficult, and we should make doctors and nurses feel grateful to us for providing them with work and pay. Regardless of their conditions of work being less than perfect, we must encourage them to 'get on with it' (something they have claimed to have been good at since the Second World War).

The way we managed the COVID-19 pandemic did not help our public image, but our COVID-19 vaccination program did. We showed a poor grip of the situation, and some managerial ineptitude. We should have given the public clearer and more consistent messages. Despite this, the public accepts that without us, our nation would have suffered more than it did. We must prepare, however, for many negative retrospective analyses of how we handled the COVID-19 pandemic. Hopefully, other crises will help to marginalise these issues. Newly emerging COVID-19 mutants should do this.

In order to assure continuing faith in our bureaucratic control, it would help if we reprimanded dissident doctors and nurses in public, and forced them to comply. The CQC must therefore regularly inspect their medical services and more aggressively seek noncompliance. It will help keep them respectful, oppressed, and under our control.

Those who control drugs should expand their work in order to punish errant prescribing. This will require more pharmacists monitoring and reporting suspect doctors. The GMC should now punish every minor indiscretion, no matter how irrelevant clinically. It might direct them to make scapegoats (keeping doctors even more fearful of the consequences of noncompliance).

With repeated appraisals and revalidations, we can make doctors respect our corporate management ethos. Because it is not respectful of their experience and value, it will prompt dissidents to retire or change jobs. It will serve our purpose to limit their numbers and remove those who claim that medical services would be better without us.

So far we have successfully made doctors finance the CQC, the GMC, as well as their own appraisals, and revalidation. This may not be possible for much longer since the amount of financial oppression people will take has limits. Since so few doctors have objected (they remain in fear of the power we wield over them), we will continue to make them pay for now.

There is always the possibility that doctors, nurses, and their patients will revolt and try to bring about fundamental change. They may try to revive long past conditions of service and practice. If it came to it, there is little doubt that most patients would be on their side. Nurses are much less likely to revolt, especially once they have replaced GPs and are receiving higher salaries.

Older doctors are liable to spread discontent. They still hark back to 'the good old days', a time when there was minimal government interference, and less managerial control over their professional lives. With luck they will remain demoralised and disheartened by our ever-tightening corporate control. Their generous NHS pensions should soften their intent to propagate revolt among their ranks. Many will choose to retire, and that will be to our advantage. The younger ones may try to escape our political, fiscal, and managerial controls, but getting themselves together will be an exercise akin to herding cats.

Doctors will argue (as dedicated altruists) that they alone should be trusted with the clinical interests of patients. They will argue that they alone know enough to manage medical practice. They will argue strongly that they are not being justly dealt with by lawyers instead of their peers. They will argue that we force them (through the GMC and CQC) to comply by creating fixed rules from guidelines. They might demand their own medical directorate, which would diminish the power and control we have vested in the GMC. They mostly hold to the strange and unmanageable notion that each patient is different, and deserves individual clinical appraisal and care. They will fancifully contend that fixed rules and obligatory guidelines cannot apply to every patient.

We know that personalised medicine based on genetic profiling, is not far away. It will be unaffordable, and must be resisted for as long as possible. While we hold the purse strings, we remain in control. Any suggestion that doctors and nurses should have any say in such matters would spell political disaster, and would undermine our administration completely. It is expedient however not to dash their hopes completely, no matter how unrealistic they get. It serves our purpose to allow them one hope: that one day, the medical profession will regain control over its practices, and once again occupy the clinical driving seat.

If patients were to join doctors and nurses in their revolt, they might object to paying so much tax. Patients might elect to pay for their own medical care, as they once did before 1948. Freedom of choice is a dangerous thing, although undoubtedly a growing trend in all spheres of life. It engenders discontent and has a destabilising influence when curtailed. It might lead to the renewed ascendance of medical insurance companies and reduced expenditure for us. We might offload large numbers of NHS patients into the private sector. It might induce them to make private medical insurance affordable, even for low-paid workers. There is a potential drawback. Many thousands of our high-earning colleagues would lose their jobs. Many would have to relocate and revert to what they were trained for, namely the corporate management of factories.

We must continue to strengthen our numbers and tighten the grip we have on the medical profession before they try to exercise their power over us. In this, we have strong political backing. It remains in the interest of our government to foster what the British public perceives as an unparalleled health service, free at the point of service.

We must endeavour to make the public realise where their trust should rest. For far too long, the public has trusted medical professionals, with doctors and nurses persistently claiming that they alone have the knowledge to manage the life and death of patients and that all medical care must become patient-centred. These ideas are not to be tolerated.

The Health Ministry. London. UK. (Dictated, but not signed).

The Politics of Medical Regulation

The regulation of the medical profession is not a fascinating subject, but it is one that no doctor or nurse can afford to ignore. Lawyers, not doctors, regulate the UK medical profession; corporate directors and managers, not clinicians, run the NHS. Medical bureaucracy tacitly insists that criticism of the NHS is tantamount to treason. As a sacred cow, the NHS requires protection. Being free at the point of service allows the cow some sanctimony. This sacred cow has priority, so patients and medical staff must take second place.

To understand what the UK medical profession has lost while in the hands of politicians, you must try to imagine the clinical freedom I once had in the 1960s. If you turned the clock back fifty years, you would at once experience more freedom to practise the art and science of medicine, relieve suffering, prevent disease, and save lives without bureaucratic control.

Corporate Folly

Corporatisation has its dangers for patients and doctors. Since the nationalisation of UK medicine in 1948, many have surfaced. Corporate medical bureaucrats demonstrate Parkinson's Law: their work constantly expands to fill the time available. Medical bureaucrats, by studying business administration, have achieved what Parkinson predicted. In the preface of his book: '*Parkinson's Law or the Pursuit of Progress*' (1958, published by John Murray), C. Northcote Parkinson wrote:

> '*Heaven forbid that students should cease to read books on the science of public or business administration provided only that these works are classified as fiction . . . Placed . . . among works of reference, they can do more damage than might at first seem possible.*'

Many other observations made by Parkinson have been realised by medical bureaucracy:

> *'It is manifest that there need be little or no relationship between the work to be done and the size of the staff to which it may be assigned.' Also: 'The number of the officials and the quantity of work are not related to each other at all.'*

Parkinson also wrote that

> *'An official wants to multiply sub-ordinates, not rivals' and 'Officials make work for each other.'*

None of these apply to doctors or nurses.

Before I qualified in 1966, an expanding army of bureaucrats had already grown to govern nurses and doctors in the UK. With the statutory powers given to them, they started to ignore our professional opinions, and slowly came to disrespect our medical sovereignty over clinical practice.

In their book *Machiavellian Intelligence,* (LID Publishing, 2018), Dr. Mark Powell and Jonathon Gifford discuss the core realities of every corporate machine. They contend that they are not social structures but instead are feudal, constantly on a war footing, having courts replete with their own etiquette and intrigues. The successful are always seeking advancement, and need loyal supporters. A corporation is a place where nobody is trusted and everyone is disposable.

The corporate insistence on standardisation dispenses with individual considerations. Instead, the rules and regulations planned to control the actions of employees are imposed universally. Standardisation is a blunt management instrument when applied to diverse and variable entities, and what entities are more diverse than patients, doctors, and their practices?

No standard, off-the-peg uniform will fit an individual

like one made to measure, except by chance. The NHS cannot afford to promote personalised doctor patient relationships, so it intends to introduce individual genomic studies in its place. This will not replace doctors practising the art of medicine or the personal doctor patient relationships found in private practice. Genomic studies, the art of medicine and personalised doctor patient relationships should be available to all patients.

Standardisation can reduce risks. The equipment required for an operation is often the same and a lot of time can be saved by theatre nurses knowing beforehand what instruments a particular surgeon is likely to need. Using standard approaches to intervention procedures can help doctors reduce risks when they are in training and inexperienced (the NHS could not function without them). The value of standardisation can disappear when novel situations arise, and what needs to be done needs to be thought through.

Standardisation works well enough for purveyors of hamburgers, but not so well for managing human beings. There is some merit in knowing that a hamburger bought in Manchester (a few hundred yards from the GMC offices) is the same as one bought in London. There is no merit in assuming that all doctors, nurses, patients, and medical practices are the same, except for making legal processes easier for corporations like the Department of Health, the NHS, and GMC to function. At least CQC inspectors visiting my practice did sometimes allow for the differences between my private practice and NHS practices, albeit using a standard set of tick-boxes for their assessments and responses. These boxes always represented the corporate NHS viewpoint, but not always mine.

David Dighton

Interfering in the Doctor Patient Relationship

For the doctor patient relationship to be fully beneficial in any other than the simplest of cases, clinical evidence needs to be reviewed relative to the patient's condition and circumstances. This is an art. No artform, including the art of medicine, is measurable, so CQC inspectors cannot assess it with certainty, even though this often determines how well a patient is managed. Because some working for the CQC think they can measure it, I once asked an inspector to describe his ruler and how he used it. This he correctly took to be irreverence.

Instead of doctors governing their own work, tiers of bureaucrats now exist to direct them. They stand ready to go further and interfere in doctor patient relationships. The CQC have been progressively approaching this for years, and are now ready to get much more involved. The case they will make uses the same old, well-worn justification. 'It is in the public interest', and not safe when patients have only doctors and nurses to rely on. In order to get more involved, they will need to override patient confidentiality. The Information Commission told me that they had this right, although they would have to apply to a court of law for access to any confidential patient records. They see this as no problem. They have our tax revenues to play with.

The disregarded elephant in the room has a question to ask. What benefit, other than basic housekeeping management (which Florence Nightingale showed to be crucial), has medical bureaucracy brought to patient morbidity, welfare, and mortality? Can we expect an answer from research, and if not, why not?

Medical Sovereignty & the Rule of law

> '*The primary role of government is to protect its citizens.*
> *The primary function of the law is to protect individuals from one another.*
> *Who is to protect individuals from the government and the law?*
> *Where government has gone beyond its limits is in deciding to protect us from ourselves.*'
> — *Ronald Reagan.*

The rules created democratically by politicians (and enforced by bureaucrats) protect and control citizens. They safeguard citizens by creating and maintaining valuable public services, such as military forces, police and fire services, medical practices, and refuse collections. They provide a format for the normal functioning of everyday life and the maintenance of the physical infrastructure. Problems arise when bureaucrats project their power beyond this infrastructure, and tamper with the superstructure. Because power can engender the desire for more power, this happens in all societies. Those who hold this power often express it arrogantly and sometimes insolently. The provision of health and social services in the UK have both been tampered with in this way.

Louis XIV, the Sun King, once summarily dismissed

all of his advisers and bureaucrats. He remarked, 'L'état, c'est moi.' Doctors can claim no equivalent power, even though many citizens regard medical professionals as indispensable.

Socrates once asked, 'Are some citizens more valuable than others?' He classified various human souls as having an equivalent value to bronze, silver, or gold when their relative value to society is judged.

So what value should society assign to those entrusted with the lives of citizens and the quality of those lives? One must consider that the acquisition of medical skills comes with a duty, which is to use them to benefit others. The knowledge and skill required lies well beyond the ability and inclination of most citizens (only 0.28% of UK citizens are doctors; 1.1% are registered nurses).

Should doctors and nurses be allowed to assume that their work sometimes sets them above the rule of law and that they are more valuable to society than bureaucrats?

For doctors and nurses, the ability to preserve life comes with a moral duty to use it as and when it is required. The care of others, regardless of any personal, economic, or political consideration, is also a sovereign duty for anyone capable of delivering it. For the common good this duty must sometimes take precedence over all other obligations to society. Nothing takes precedence over our individual duty to protect the life and death of others. We should only be made to comply with the CQC, GMC, and PSA when what they demand is clinically appropriate. Permission for doctors and nurses to presume this right must feature in future legislation.

In 1948 Aneurin Bevan created the NHS (largely based on the Welsh, Tredegar Workmen's Medical Aid Society) not only to remove the need for patients to pay for medical services, but also to bring the UK medical profession under state control. Those doctors who dissented worried about the implications of nationalisation and the corporatisation of the medical profession. As predicted by many, doctors became politically demoted while medical bureaucrats were promoted.

For millennia doctors and nurses practiced freely, with no need for an overseeing bureaucracy (except to certificate the adequacy of our learning). Once upon a time (a few decades ago), no secretary, receptionist, or practice managers would ever have presumed to direct the work of doctors or nurses. Not so now! The bureaucracy doctors must now contend with in the UK engulfs doctors and nurses in regulations that direct their every move, often restricting the delivery of essential interventions.

Politicians know full well that the dedication doctors and nurses have to their patients prohibits them from leaving their posts, although juniors did strike for a day on the 12th January 2016, the first doctors' strike in forty years (they disputed details of a new contract). With the British Medical Association (BMA) requesting a 35% pay rise, junior doctors in the UK began a 72-hour walkout on the 13th March 2023, and went on strike for a further four days on the 11th April 2023. Completely fenced in morally, politically, and legally, the medical profession has little option but to submit to bureaucratic control. Like Louis XIV, doctors undoubtedly possess sovereignty over the lives of others, but theirs is an impotent form of political sovereignty.

Nurses went on strike for six days at the end of 2022 and again between the 30th April and the 2nd of May 2023. Pay was the issue.

In 2020-21, the status of a few medically qualified doctors

with bureaucratic roles became apparent because of their appearances on the TV during the government briefings about COVID-19. Although such work will mostly have detached them from the clinical arena, those who appeared had obviously kept a duty to preserve life on a grander scale than practising doctors. They helped steer government policy. They provided pertinent analysis and a clinical perspective to political decision makers. It would be wrong to think inductively and conclude that an equivalent usefulness applies to all medically qualified bureaucrats. The decision makers then had the unenviable job of balancing lives with the health of the economy.

Because of its critical importance to us all, the job of saving lives and relieving suffering naturally supersedes all other internal societal matters. It takes precedence over the dictates of rule-makers and regulators, unless they are engaged in keeping unruly mobs and invaders under control, thus preventing loss of life on the streets.

Patient Individuality

Patients have rights as individuals. One they do not have in the UK under the NHS is the right to choose their doctor. Another is that they cannot change their GP or seek another opinion, without their GP's permission. There are strict bureaucratic rules applied to GP practices and the patients they can add to their list.

Religious sovereignty over citizens arose in twelfth century Rome. Popes accepted a plenitude of power over souls while royalty kept sovereignty over the bodies of their subjects. With moral equality in the eyes of God, people were first seen as individuals (*Inventing the Individual.* Larry Siedentop. London, Allen Lane, 2014).

Health Metrics

There is only one good, knowledge, and one evil, ignorance.
—Socrates. Lives of Eminent Philosophers.
Diogenes Laertius (469 BC - 399 BC)

The health metrics that count the most are morbidity and mortality.

All corporations know that measures of performance will help them improve their performance. They can define improvement as more profit, greater efficiency, faster growth, improved cost-effectiveness, or greater customer satisfaction. While mostly true for retail operations, can it be true for medical practice?

During their business management studies, medical bureaucrats learn that feedback metrics can improve patient care and health outcomes. Unfortunately,there will never be reliable metrics for complex entities like quality of service and patient care. Florence Nightingale used mortality metrics to persuade the government to change medical services, and proved the value of an experienced medical observer for improving the care of patients. Most useful insights and helpful ideas in medical practice come from something simpler than anonymous data collection. That is the personal observations of those with experience. Those who thoroughly understand medical practice and what it takes to achieve high standards.

Observing workers working and customers being dealt with will reveal at a glance most of the important issues for business corporations.

Judgements based on metrics can mislead for many reasons (measuring the wrong entity, assigning the wrong significance to that entity, and summing the errors of numerical measures). They are cheap to create and employ, however, and best suit those with little experience and understanding, and those who wish to keep their distance (like NHS executives).

Do we need more data, or just a few key data points to understand better? The acquisition and valuing of anonymous data now drives many big data projects. The idea is this: if only we can analyse enough data thoroughly, valuable discoveries will surely emerge. The idea has caught the imagination of many corporations. The hope is that it will allow them to continue to control anonymously, when in reality it has always been personal commitment and hands-on involvement that drives the most successful businesses. Unfortunately the belief in anonymous big data has led medical bureaucracy to requisition and collect more and more data. With resources forever limited, this pursuit must surely have reduced the finance available for patient care.

There are many instances in science where data collected before and after an intervention has led to genuine insights and progress. Regardless of how many repeated anecdotal observations reliable observers make, we should always use some independent metric for confirmation. For scientists such evidence is essential when trying to prove something new. Unfortunately many of the metrics doctors and nurses now keep for regulators are of no clinical significance. If medical staff were once racehorses, they are now used as carthorses! I would have no objection to managerial metrics if regulators employed their own staff to collect them. The only metrics needed are those that lead to improvements in morbidity and mortality.

Socrates thought ignorance evil, but there is a greater crime: allowing oneself to be led by the ignorant, given that intelligence, experience, and education are readily available. Ignorance is everywhere, and there is not a bureaucratic monopoly. Ignorance of ignorance is now endemic in every society and growing in popularity. The medical profession commits a serious collective crime against patients when it allows those with little or no medical knowledge to control how they practice medicine.

We now live in an age where those empowered by the myth of intellectual equality and knowledge gleaned from the internet can hold as many fanciful medical ideas and opinions as they like and broadcast them on social media. Although we are all witnessing information overload (most of the information sent to us is irrelevant), understanding is diminishing as technology becomes more arcane.

Professional Disgrace and Medical Bureaucracy

Apart from knowing about business and corporate management, what can medical bureaucrats hope to bring to a forum, composed of experienced doctors and nurses discussing clinical cases? Instead of benefit, might they not bring harm? The following examples suggest that a fear of bureaucracy can be justified.

WARNING TO READERS:
What follows could prove shocking.

The Case of Jack Adcock

Six-year-old Jack Adcock and his parents were victims of inadequate care in the NHS. Dr. Bawa-Garba, a junior paediatrician in training, was considered solely responsible for what happened to Jack in 2011. But was she?

The GMC thought Dr. Bawa-Garba solely responsible even though (a) those supervising her were unavailable (no senior doctor helped her interpret high blood lactate levels, or confirmed the diagnosis of sepsis), and (b) NHS management was deficient (staff shortages, and a nonfunctioning hospital computer system - evidence not presented in court). Perhaps of most significance was the undoubted misdirection of another doctor on duty (not Dr Bawa-Garba), who agreed to Jack's mother's suggestion that he should take his usual enalapril medication, given that he had improved somewhat (he had Down's syndrome, and heart disease). He subsequently went into cardiac arrest and did not recover.

To give enalapril (blood pressure treatment) to an already hypotensive patient with sepsis must rank amongst the worst of all therapeutic decisions.

Having been convicted of manslaughter, Dr. Bawa-Garba was struck off the medical register (the High Court granted the GMC permission to overturn the MPTS decision to keep her on the medical register. They can no longer do this). She became a single parent without a job.

The heartless damage wrought to Dr. Bawa-Garba's personal life and circumstances as a result was horrendous. A few years later, on the 13th of August 2018, the High Court ruling was overturned. With the help of crowdfunding, and a review of her case, she became re-instated as a GMC registered doctor.

The case of Dr. Hediza Bawa-Garba allows insight into the anatomy and functioning of the MPTS/GMC's legal bureaucratic power. It illustrates the disproportionate, inappropriate, and disrespectful damage that can be inflicted on a doctor in training, when the blame more justly belonged to hospital administrators and the senior colleagues who left her abandoned.

The Case of Surgeon Mr. David Sellu

Experienced surgeon Mr. David Sellu, with forty years of operating experience, and no complaints against him, had to deal with an urgent case of faecal peritonitis (February 2010). He could find no available anaesthetist, or get urgent access to an operating theatre while working in a private hospital. After he eventually operated, the patient later died of septicaemia. For his part in the affair, they charged Mr Sellu with gross negligence and manslaughter.

Sellu served a prison sentence following a Coroner's Inquest and police action (*Did He Save Lives?* David Sellu. Sweetcroft Publishing, 2019). On November 15th 2016, three judges at the Royal Courts of Justice quashed his previous conviction. He later appeared at an MPTS hearing, at which they declared him clear of all unfit practices, and restored him to the medical register.

Mr. Sellu received no respect for the many lives he had saved while dutifully upkeeping his sovereign clinical role. He was clearly an experienced, successful surgeon, with considerable ability. I have little doubt that with full exposure of the facts (much administrative detail remained undeclared), few doctors would have regarded his part in the patient's death as a crime. The object of the legal action against him was simple. It was to remove a criminal from lifesaving work, thereby risking more deaths than the one in question.

In both cases, the medical profession commented (in the BMJ and on Twitter, etc.) but remained ineffective. There was no widespread exposure to public opinion, and therefore no display of common sense. While trying to reach their own internal targets for convictions, legal and medical bureaucratic organisations can inflict malicious damage on those dedicated to saving lives simply as a matter of course. After all, every faceless corporation has an absolute requirement: every employee must follow orders (mindless or otherwise). What makes such scenarios even more sinister is that our system of regulatory bureaucracy and those who serve it have nothing to lose personally.

All doctors recognise the rightful role of the GMC to investigate, and to remove criminal doctors who callously harm patients. Many doctors, however, now regard the GMC as a fearsome legal adversary, pursuing a culture of oppression, blame, and retribution, with no understanding of clinical practice. Like racism in the Metropolitan Police force, these are intrinsic to their established culture. The GMC has the temerity to believe that their tribunals and their third-party referees can assess the clinical risks doctors take every day, as well as the risks that specific doctors present to patients. How can any legally based corporate system possibly claim sufficient qualification and clinical understanding to make risk assessments safely, given no knowledge of medical practice, or of the doctor on trial, other than that available as recorded evidence?

When performing their statutory role, the GMC and others can present a danger to both the public and the medical profession. Many excellent doctors and nurses dedicated to the care of their patients have become disenchanted and demoralised with their corporate bureaucracy. Many have left the profession, emigrated, or are giving serious thought to leaving the medical profession. The attrition rate amongst doctors in training is growing fast.

During the period under review (2005–2013), there were twenty-eight reported cases of suicide among doctors undergoing GMC investigation procedures. *GMC Internal Review (2014)*: Sarndrah Horsfal, Independent Consultant.

Those of us who are old enough, and who are secure enough at the time, can easily opt out and retire, leaving these oppressive legalistic goings-on behind us. This is not an option younger doctors and nurses should need to take.

The collective loss of knowledge and experience caused by alienating doctors is inestimable, but then how can we reasonably expect any medical legislator, regulator, or bureaucrat to respect the medical knowledge we have or the value of our personal clinical experience? After working for a few years in an office full of medical bureaucrats, I can say that many of them despised doctors, rather than respecting them. This is part of their inculcated culture handed down from one to another.

Of far less significance than the cases described were my own clashes with the GMC. Two pharmacists reported me to the GMC, without them discussing my clinical reasoning with me. As in the case of David Sellu, I have little doubt that all these instances would have been regarded as minor by doctors with decades of prescribing experience and knowledge of how the treatment requirements of individual patients can vary and present challenges (my patient remained safe in my care for over 6 years, despite what two pharmacists and the MPTS thought to be my dangerous prescribing).

An MPTS tribunal, composed of a lawyer, a biologist, and a Birmingham GP (with half of my experience), thought I lacked the experience necessary to prescribe controlled drugs. They also thought I lacked insight into the clinical risks. They thought I would be a danger to patients in the future (after fifty-three years of taking significant clinical risks as an interventional cardiologist and general physician, and after doing no harm). In November 2020 they suspended me for one year. In response, I retired (aged 76). After one year, a High Court granted the PSA the right to command the GMC to strike me off the medical register (though they had agreed to my voluntary retirement); they did not want me returning to practice. (Read more details and comments in Appendices 1 & 2).

The PSA summary of their case against me and the GMC makes for interesting reading (Appendix 2). Can you guess the real reasons behind their action? Did my disrespect for their regulatory processes concern them most? They thought my (supposed) lack of clinical insight (lawyers know all about this, of course), meant that there was little chance I would mend my ways and bend to their higher wisdom.

There is a serious fundamental problem with all these regulatory GMC processes. Lawyers, and mostly GPs (because they are more readily available) are the ones assessing clinical risk. Few of them could profess to be qualified for this key judgement since GPs refer any case that might be risky to hospital doctors.

On the same spectrum of dismissive disrespect handed down by the GMC, MPTS, PSA, and CPS mentioned above, comes the CQC. The CQC has a valuable job to do. The safety of hospitals and medical premises do need regular review, but by whom? Their inspecting teams often include medical and nursing experts but that need not continue after they become restricted to evaluating housekeeping matters.

The CQC can overstep the mark when, as a legal corporation, they interfere in doctor patient relationships, rather than housekeeping and building safety issues. In keeping with other medical regulatory authorities, they will probably label any doctor or nurse who shows them disrespect a 'troublemaker' or 'dissenter' (Dr. H. Beerstecher, for instance. See below). Once so marked, the dissenters will be spied on, and repeatedly visited,to detect further evidence of their noncompliance. The aim is to bring offenders 'into line'. I found their attitudes and actions inconsistent with the level of respect afforded by patients to those who can save their lives and help improve their health. Inappropriate disrespect of one group for another can be endemic, and can be rooted out only by a complete change of culture. That will mean changing all the staff and the regime.

If you think what I have written so far about regulatory agencies is far-fetched and paranoid, consider the fate of one doctor who dared to challenge the sanctimony of CQC inspectors.

The Beerstecher Intervention

In 2016, Dr. Hendrik Beerstecher secretly filmed his CQC inspection. The CQC inspectors felt this to be an unfair intrusion on their privacy (at my practice, they always held discussions behind closed doors). His aim was to allow others to judge for themselves whether the watchdog had made inaccurate judgments of his practice.

In March 2018 the MPTS suspended Dr. Beerstecher for two months after he accused the CQC of 'boohoo', 'secrets', and an 'orchestrated smear'. He published videos of his inspection on YouTube without the CQC's permission. By suspending him without further notice, the MPTS left all his patients in the lurch without a GP, and unable to find another one quickly enough for safety. So much for their concern for public safety.

The MPTS thought that Dr. Beerstecher's actions would have 'a negative impact on both patients and confidence in the medical profession'. Really? On what evidence? His comments would have simply reinforced the opinion held by many doctors, and confirmed the opinions of most of my patients: (1) that regulators have too much power, (2) they are too full of their own importance (compared to doctors), and (3) they interfere, despite having far less medical knowledge and knowhow than doctors.

There is a key question. Who should the public trust more with their medical care: legally oriented, management trained, corporate medical bureaucrats, or practising doctors?

This was not the end of the matter for Dr. Beerstecher. Since all regulatory bodies support one another they will join forces against whosoever they see as an adversary. Those responsible for the NHS provision of his practice closed it down. They obviously knew that at his age, and with a suspension on his record, he would not easily find another job as an NHS GP. Collectively they denied many patients the valued experience of the doctor they knew and trusted. CQC inspectors clearly had their pride bruised. As a result, they ignored every consideration of immediate patient care, patient continuity, and patient choice. They did, however, provide us with a good example of the insolence of power.

I wonder how many patients have lost their lives or suffered because of doctors being sanctioned, suspended, or removed? Do medical bureaucrats care? They are just doing their job, and can always incite the Nuremberg defence: 'I was only following orders!'

As a postscript to the Beerstecher case, Wimbledon GP Dr. Paul Cundy recommended that GPs should make recordings of CQC inspections in order to gain evidence for any complaints that might arise. He did not suggest the recordings should be covert.

Ruth Rankine, CQC Deputy Inspector of general practice who studied business, French and Spanish for her BA, rather than medicine, said (as reported by *Pulse* magazine) that their inspection teams should be able to do their job without experiencing this type of treatment from medical professionals. She clearly holds the view that CQC inspectors have a status equal or superior to that of experienced doctors, engaged in saving lives and relieving suffering. From whence comes such sanctimony? It is part of the bureaucratic culture, the assumption being that their work is essential, and that the plight of patients would be so much worse without them.

The CQC should take time to consider how their inspectors function. Are they justified in suggesting any form of superiority? Instead of being earnest about corporate audits, they might take time to consider what real, day-to-day medicine entails, and why it is so valued by millions. If patients value their doctor, the CQC should attempt to learn why. They should come to learn and discuss, and not to preach and enforce. They should learn to appreciate doctors, and offer them positive help rather than create problems that are a hindrance. They may have the law on their side, but that does not justify their often high-handed attitude, least of all towards those with so much more experience and superior knowledge of medical practice. For millennia we have trained doctors to deliver medical care without the interference of bureaucrats and, like Dr. Hendrik Beerstecher and myself, without significant complaints from patients.

The elephant in the discussion room has a few questions to ask. What was it about the behaviour of these and previous CQC inspectors, that moved Dr. Beerstecher to act as he did? Is there ever smoke without fire? How many CQC inspectors have the medical knowledge to match his, or that of any other doctor they inspect? How many inspectors get to know patients as well as their GP? How many CQC inspectors really appreciate the experience and talent required to deal with hundreds of patients over long periods without complaint?

All CQC inspectors wear badges of authority, but in matters of human welfare and medical care, humanity should be given precedence. Their employment contracts should reflect this.

Few questioned the precedence given to doctors and nurses

during the COVID-19 pandemic. So why not at other times? The rules governing the CCQ should be made to respect the medical sovereignty held by doctors and nurses. One reason is that they simply cannot do what doctors and nurses do. In claiming to occupy the moral high ground, bureaucrats have lost direction. Their attitudes need to be reset in line with the primacy most societies give to doctors and nurses.

Instead of sanctimony, the CQC should try humility. Like all those who seek the truth, they too should research the validity of their opinions and directives. They could have undertaken an audit of Dr. Beerstecher's patients, (a) to see what they thought about CQC inspections, and their usefulness, and (b) to find out how much they valued him as a doctor. Patients are the ones who vote for political authority, and we need to engage them to challenge the assumptions held by medical regulators, the most onerous of which is that they alone are knowledgeable enough to safeguard medical practice and patient safety. Statute law empowers the CQC, GMC, and PSA, so political and legal change would have to occur before any regulator will change. Changing their culture will be more difficult.

Is Patient Confidentiality a Fiasco?

The CQC can inspect patients' notes, regardless of any information protection afforded by the Information Commission. They can do this under the Health and Social Care Act 2008. Article 6, (e) of GDPR legislation also allows for it (when in 'the public interest'). They can countermand any confidentiality rights doctors and patients think they have by getting a High Court judge to enforce their wishes. Just to remind you, I am not discussing the behaviour of a Fascist regime, an autocracy, or an oligarchy.

So, what trust can patients have in doctor patient confidentiality when regulators have such powers? Should we trust them unconditionally when they wave their badges of authority at us? They think so. My experiences with them have led me to conclude that the safest strategy is to regard all government agencies as enemies. You will then fare better when called to deal with them. They all insist that you can trust them, and that it would be better to cooperate. Where have I heard that before? My advice is to never give them the impression that you are an innocent, like 'Little Red Riding Hood'.

As I know from personal experience, the CQC allows spying on doctors. Instead of doing the underhand work themselves, they employ 'stakeholders' (spying agencies). They can telephone, pretending to be patients, in order to find evidence against your practice. Doctors will regard this as paranoia at their peril.

One of my patients who had no personal complaint against me objected to the CQC delving into her treatment records without her consent or mine. The Information Commission told me that the CQC are allowed to access any clinical notes they want, even if the patient disagreed. A High Court will accept that any government agency wanting patient information will be doing so 'in the public interest'. Medical confidentiality is thus a fiasco. Another patient of mine, an ex-nurse, was told directly by the GMC, 'it doesn't matter whether you give your consent, we will get all your clinical notes from Dr. Dighton, whenever we wish.' Their justification was that 'all dangerous and criminal doctors must be purged.' The implication: 'any loss of confidentiality is of secondary importance.'

A-Level students intending to become medical students might like to write an essay: 'Compare and contrast what I have described with the tactics advised by Machiavelli, and how Fascist and totalitarian states behave.'

On one occasion in October 2018, a high-handed, medically qualified CQC inspector (a lecturer in General Practice) demonstrated his arrogance and open disrespect for me and my practice. Dr. Beerstecher had perhaps experienced something similar. He walked into my patient notes room without my permission (I had all A4 folder notes at the time), and began pulling out notes for inspection. I wrote to all the patients concerned, and all strongly objected, but only after the event.

This CQC GP inspector referred the contents of some of my patient notes to the GMC for their further evaluation (I had no NHS overseers). He thought a general physician should not function as a GP (I had no appropriate certification for the most elementary form of medical practice). At the time of my inspection, I argued the clinical case for each patient (from the point of view of having been a lecturer in hospital medicine and cardiology), but he was not open to any academic medical discussion. Instead he displayed his unfortunate nature: that of a single-minded, bigoted corporate drone. It is true, I had no current certificate for 'NHS general practice' (I practiced what I thought was general medicine, having last been a partner GP in 1971). This upset him most. 'General Practice is now a specialty,' he proclaimed. He must have thought I lacked the know-how to use an oroscope or diagnose tonsillitis and varicose veins. It is, of course, widely accepted that one cannot perform anything safely without a valid certificate!

Some forms of accreditation are essential, especially in the invasive specialties we choose to practise, like cardiology and surgery. If they can show that properly evaluated certification protects the public, who would disagree?

To function as a GP in my early days as a doctor, all I required was an elementary knowledge of medicine, surgery, and gynaecology/obstetrics. One would never have dared compare that level of knowledge to that of hospital physicians, surgeons, and gynaecologists. So what has changed?

After this incident with the CQC, I ceased all consultations for minor ailments (GP work, by definition). Many hundreds of patients wrote letters to me expressing their disappointment. They had no NHS GP, and had no wish to have one. The reason they consulted me in the first place was to get more time, consideration, expertise, and experience than was on offer in NHS general practices. I was a GP Principal in 1968 and stayed in-post until intense boredom overcame me. I happily resigned the role to become a cardiac research fellow.

The GP CQC inspector I mentioned before was right about one thing: the bureaucracy attached to GP practice, and its management has moved on. It is now bound by so much red tape that GPs need to specialise in handling it. Patients' medical needs have, of course, not changed. These incidents lacked both clinical and common sense.

On a subsequent inspection, I told the CQC inspectors that they could not view my clinical notes, and if they insisted, I would ask them to leave. My point was that data protection matters, at least to me and my patients. I was not about to compromise patient confidentiality again. Having reminded me of their legal standing and authority, their immediate reaction was to show me their badges of authority. I told them to address all their legal protestations to my lawyers. I suggested

I would stick to practising medicine if they stuck to their corporate business.

I had, of course, anticipated their demands and reactions (rule-based people are entirely predictable). I had copied the notes of my last ten patients, with all identifiers removed. They ungraciously accepted my *fait accompli*, rather than have to leave with their tails between their legs. From that point on, my card will have been marked. Once they have identified a dissident doctor, they will take every opportunity to hassle and remove him, an old political strategy that remains alive and well. Do not act as I did unless, like me, you are old (I was seventy years of age at the time). By then, most antiestablishmentarians will feel free to speak their mind.

Death, Bureaucracy and Clinical Management Freedom

Many decades ago, amphetamines were thought to be wonder drugs. Only our perception has changed. They are still wonder drugs! Be prepared to examine any pharmaceutical biases you might have (and the dictates of medical bureaucracy), and favour some objective facts. Amphetamines improve arousal, depression, vitality, and drive; they improve motivation, energy, and happiness, and cause no organ damage (unlike alcohol and tobacco). They are also addictive and, like alcohol, dangerous in overdose.

Some of the commonest species of bureaucrat Homo utopiensis are committed to creating a drug-free society. Their aim is to stamp out addiction, regardless of any clinical or social benefit. Financially secure, middle-class bureaucrats will struggle to understand the plight of the poor and deprived. They will thus reject any need for an addiction (alcohol, cannabis, and benzodiazepines) which might help some tolerate their plight. While politicians and their bureaucrats cannot remove poverty, they will try their best to remove anything that might ease its sufferance.

Utopia is a place where all are happy, addiction-free, and content with the world created for them by bureaucrats. Everyone there has a fulfilled, comfortable life. Both inside and outside of the walls of Utopia, medical bureaucrats enjoy the power to descend on any doctor who dares to prescribe an addictive drug, whatever might be its advantages to some. If we accept the delusion of Utopia, why not go further and ignore the fact that tobacco and alcohol cause considerable mortality, yet remain legal? Many enjoy them both, but suffer considerable consequences. Why, then, ignore the happiness and contentment some achieve while using physically harmless but addictive pharmaceuticals like benzodiazepines, analgesics, and some stimulants? Having been given the task of protecting the public, how can medical bureaucrats maintain their hypocritical position while ignoring clinical experience?

Should we feel sorry for all bureaucrats living in a lax, underregulated world, one which constantly criticises their imposition of rules? One must appreciate the difficulty they have living in a world where patients want freedom from oppression, and trust doctors more than government officials. A world where patients trust doctors to know most about the drugs they prescribe.

Perhaps I have it all wrong? I thought the aim of doctors and nurses was to make patients' lives more tolerable. Obviously I lack the insight to know better! More discipline might be the answer. Disrespectful maverick that I am, I have always found it difficult to accept adherence to bureaucratic rules that conflict with my patient's welfare. It must be my age! If I had not retired from complying with bureaucratic nonsense when I did, perhaps a few corrective training courses and more appraisals and revalidations, would have rescued me from further corporate dissent? I might have realised just how lucky I was to have been guided by so many dedicated, wise medical bureaucrats. Without them, my patients might have remained exposed to a doctor motivated to inflict harm on them while stealing their cash.

Nonsense, like truth, does has a certain ring to it, don't you think?

The medical disasters and mishaps that occur in NHS hospitals and GP practices each year in the UK suggest that major harm to patients flows directly from medical bureaucracy. Consider the case of my patient, Ms. Eva Wade.

Eva was an intelligent Hungarian librarian, who had tried all the usual anti-depressants available in the 1990s, without benefit. Both her father and grandfather had suffered the same condition decades earlier, in the 1930s and 1940s. In their day, they had benefitted appreciably from amphetamine (a euphoric, if not an anti-depressant). I had never known a patient offered an amphetamine for depression (for bureaucratic, not pharmacological reasons), so some research was necessary.

Having done that research, and having found no known side-effects from small doses, I let her have a one-week trial of amphetamine 5mgs twice daily. Addiction, albeit to a physically harmless drug, was bound to occur. But would addiction be a greater problem to her than depression? The result was a little less than amazing. It improved her motivation, rather than reducing it (a common effect of some antidepressants). While

140

taking amphetamine, she found the energy to change all her depressing life circumstances.

Using the same tactic developed by the Tokubetsu Kōgekitai (Japanese Special Attack Unit), otherwise known as kamikaze, two inspectors from the local Controlled Drugs Agency (CDA) in Epping, Essex (one was a GP) descended on my practice.

The object of their visit was to gather evidence for my being a danger to the public, a dangerous drug-pusher, posing as a doctor. They lodged a report with the GMC, who presumably recorded me as a dangerous, singlehanded private doctor, an out-of-control drug pusher lacking insight into the consequences of his actions. The incident gave them reason to look further and search for other evidence of my prescribing misdemeanours. But that came later. I had to tell Eva that I could not continue prescribing amphetamine sulphate for her, despite its unexpectedly successful effects. Perhaps we could find a psychiatrist to continue it, given its obvious efficacy (not a concept considered by the bureaucrat CDA officials, whose insistence on compliance forsook clinical judgement)?

After Eva committed suicide several weeks later, I wrote to the CDA with an indefensible allegation. I accused them of being (indirectly) responsible for her death. Words are sometimes mightier than the sword, and those empowered to interfere with patient management should know the consequences of their actions, and be made responsible for them. The Nuremburg defence of just 'doing their duty' cut no mustard with me. The directives of the bureaucrats who visited me had brought about the death of my patient.

I have always wondered how my visitors from the CDA have lived, knowing the result of their intervention. Strangely those who espouse feedback, like the many bureaucrats doctors have to deal with remained silent. My comments were, of course, logged with the CDA, CQC, and GMC, ready for use against me whenever expedient. That's the way regulators work. I hoped my comments would provide them with some useful educational clinical material should they ever wish to consider the consequences of their actions while protecting the public. Their sanctimony would not normally allow it, of course.

I thought sacrificing the few for the many was for Commanders-in-Chief (like Churchill and Eisenhower, in the Second World War), not for subordinate office workers. In fact, no corporate committee, whether within the CDA, GMC, or CQC, need consider the clinical consequences of their actions. As enforcers of weaponised rules (guidelines made immutable), this is not a job requirement. Striving for a Utopian world, but isolated from the realities faced each day by our patients, it is easy for them to remain happily deluded. It is also easy for them to remain content hiding behind their legalised metaphysical missions 'to protect the public (from doctors)' and 'to prevent the medical profession from falling into disrepute'. Nothing here about positively benefitting doctors and their patients, you notice.

The public are mostly unaware of the dangers we all face from medical and government bureaucracy (if Dominic Cummings' allegations of 2021 were correct). It is usually only when scandal surfaces, as in the Bawa-Garba case, that the public gets a glimpse of what doctors suffer at the hand of bureaucracy.

Only doctors experienced enough for clinical judgement should decide what is best for patients. Who better than their doctor to decide who is a typical therapeutic case (for whom published guidelines are applicable), and who is an exceptional case (given their particular, atypical, clinical circumstances, as in the case of Eva Wade)? This freedom no longer exists for doctors in the UK.

Compliance Management

In a UK medical profession ruled by bureaucrats, universal compliance to their corporate values and protocols is now essential for all nurses and doctors. They might thus avoid suffering career changing retribution.

The rise of medical bureaucratic power has had many negative consequences for patients. Standardisation in delivery of corporate services may satisfy average demand, but what happens to the exceptional cases at either end of the distribution spectrum who are far from average? Standardisation can disadvantage them, and even lead to their death. Bureaucrats have had to suppress patient individuality and devalue medical judgement in order to function. Their culture, which embodies the attempt to suppress individuality (by serving only average cases) is running out of road, given that genomic studies will soon define it completely. Understanding individuality is the Holy Grail of medical assessment and deciding on treatment. This will be genome-based, personalised medicine. Where will the 'one size fits all' standardisation of bureaucratic control be then?

Although they may be slow to change, and can provide only sparse proof of their benefit to patients in the UK, I am confident that collectively they are smart enough to survive. They can then continue to punish an already ailing medical profession.

'Good Medical Practice': A Useful Guide or Legal Instrument?

The GMC's 'Good Medical Practice' is a worthy document from which no sentient and experienced health care worker will learn much. Those who regard its contents as instructive could be inexperienced or in the wrong job. As good as it is in commonsense terms, one can hardly expect it to convert an incompetent doctor into a competent one. It is much more likely to help noncompliant doctors (if ignorant of the rules) to become compliant. The GMC uses it as a standard legal instrument when assessing doctors' performance.

'Good Medical Practice' directs us to be *'polite and considerate'* to patients, and to *'treat patients as individuals'*. Were these instructions written for doctors or lawyers? I am unsure. Those who would benefit from such platitudes must be seriously deficient in the basic interpersonal skills needed to practise medicine. But that is to miss the point. These platitudes are the GMC's reference standard, dictating how doctors should practice and avoid allegations of noncompliance.

Is there another point to these directives, other than to establish the lowest possible baseline for medical professional behaviour? The text hardly functions as an instrument of guidance for anyone intelligent and sensitive enough to function as a successful doctor. Perhaps the NHS needs such guidance given how frequently an insensitive mode of behaviour is in evidence there? No private practice would survive financially without this guidance being the minimal requirement

Are these the standards required to guide less than suitable students being accepted into medical schools, later to be employed by the NHS? I doubt it, but it is a possibility! Might private medical schools groom their students differently? Nearer to the truth, I suspect, is that *'Good Medical Practice'* serves to define compliant behaviour for those lawyers who prosecute doctors, and as a beginner's guide for NHS doctors.

By allowing *'Good Medical Practice'* to set the bar so low, even minor incidents of noncompliance could trap doctors and nurses in litigation.

As binary legal instruments go, each statement in *'Good Medical Practice'* will define the behaviour expected for compliance. Wise decision-making must always include metainformation, yet the GMC (MPTS) may choose not to include it when judging allegations against doctors. I was told that taking my patient's views into account was hearsay. If they wish, they can ignore the specific circumstances of each patient and doctor, his track-record, his experience, and the patient's personal and clinical characteristics. The third-party doctors they employ as expert referees do not need to consider the doctor, his patients as individuals, or his individual circumstances. They are also directed to regard metainformation as hearsay.

Few tribunals composed of a lawyer, a layperson, and an NHS GP (a common format for an MPTS tribunal) will be qualified to judge a doctor's clinical judgements and decisions. They have statutory authority, but will not always appropriate clinical expertise. They depend only on *'Good Medical Practice'*, the *BNF* and NICE guidelines in clinical matters. Using these as the only reference points (albeit the very best scientific evidence on offer) they can make judgements that can be life changing for doctors and their practices, even when no patient complained or suffered (as in my case). The medically inexpert composition of such tribunals makes their consideration of clinical issues unsafe. In clinical matters, the MPTS section of the GMC needs to be replaced by a tribunal composed only of appropriately experienced doctors. It is right that we give laypeople and patients a voice, but not a vote.

Medical Regulators as Adversaries

The GMC is an adversarial, legally based corporation, not an academic medical organisation, yet it is empowered to investigate all clinical allegations against doctors.

MPTS tribunal members are hardly qualified to discuss more than basic medical concepts and clinical practices. I cannot question their legal perspective, but their clinical perspective would hardly stand up to academic challenges. They are in the same position as a medical student 'fresher' attending an advanced medical conference. They might pick up a few clues about the topics being discussed, but will not fully comprehend the clinical perspective. In my case only the NHS GP tribunal member was in any way qualified to discuss medical science or any aspect of the art of medicine. Had he any inclination to understand why I handled my cases as I did, he would have questioned me accordingly. He did not. Their job was simply to decide whether their rules and regulations had been broken, and (in their opinion) with what amount of disregard or recklessness.

One crucial duty they have on behalf of the public, is to guess what future risk a doctor will present to patients. How can they be comfortable doing that with no clinical perspective, other than that provided by third-party doctors, trained as independent medical referees? It is only because they too see their job as part of a legal process, and not a medical one. The medical referees they employ are not always clinically active physicians and surgeons who deal with clinical risk. GPs are naturally anxious about sick patients, and must delegate them to hospital doctors. Despite their minimal acquaintance with clinical risk taking, it will be a GP who will most likely be the medical representative on an MPTS tribunal. Any MPTS assessment of clinical risk must thus rest on guesswork, since we cannot expect a lawyer, a layperson, and a GP to always appreciate the actual clinical risks involved.

Unfortunately for any doctor appearing before them, every MPTS tribunal in doubt (and they must often be in doubt with insufficient clinical knowledge) will need to act in a failsafe way. This will naturally move them to overestimate clinical risk, even if unjust suspensions and removals from the medical register result. They must be comfortable with scapegoats, and must protect themselves at all costs.

Unless they reject a case at an early stage through lack of evidence, an adversarial contest between barristers will follow. This is the process by which the MPTS tries allegations. In this adversarial game, one barrister will try to paint the plaintiff in virtuous white, and the other will try to paint her in demonic black. This contest does not resemble any scientific discussion I have experienced. If truth requires Technicolor to portray it, the evidence served up in courts, painted only in black and white, will not always do the picture justice. For the sake of clarity, and the limited understanding of tribunal members, the entire legal process must crystallise medical practices into *reductio ad absurdum.*

Their ill-defined, metaphysical duty to 'protect the

public' from doctors and nurses allows regulators the power to instigate any form of enquiry they like (including witch-hunts). In line with all other enforcement and policing agency, any infringement they suspect could get attached to your name. You can then be flagged up and followed up in the future whenever it is deemed necessary (by an anonymous bureaucrat). Their authority allows them a plenitude of reasons for surveillance, justified by their favourite mantra: 'in the public interest'. The duty of every government is to protect the public, it's what we pay them for! The question is, are they qualified for the job?

Once they believe that they have proven an allegation against you, pharmacists, the GMC, the CQC, the PSA, and the public will be notified of a potentially dangerous renegade doctor in their midst. They will publish their views about you on the internet, so anyone searching on your name will get access to all their judgements and comments, but none of yours. They have the IT power to make sure that their postings reach the top of every Google search. Yours will be given nothing like the same preference.

If your mind has wandered, and you thought I was describing the Stasi, the former Hungarian ÁVH, or some other secret policing organisation, you would be mistaken!

What is the point of all this? It is to warn doctors of the consequences of engaging the displeasure of medical bureaucrats. Many of my wiser colleagues working for the NHS have known all about this since they qualified; they obviously knew better than me how to keep their heads below the parapet. Russian citizens quickly learned to do the same when the KGB was active; East Germans learned how to avoid Stasi witch-hunts, but should UK doctors really have to fear medical regulators in the same way?

Taken together, medical regulators can deem it their duty (in the public interest) to act against you. Like Julius Caesar, attacked by a group of 'friends', there will be little you can do against a group of self-righteous, rulebook-waving officials. Unlike Caesar's 'friends, Romans and countrymen', they carry only metaphorical knives! Any comparison to Julius Caesar is inaccurate. Caesar had much more chance of surviving his 'friends' than you will have of surviving a gang of antipathetic medical bureaucrats. They will try their best not to honour and inter any good you have done.

All doctors and nurses should take heart. Bureaucratic spite is no match for the high regard many patients will have of you. Few bureaucrats (if any) have ever been so honoured. In each of their fields of work, many of your patients will have encountered parallel examples of bureaucratic nonsense and vindictiveness, and will readily take your side.

Perhaps what I have written is paranoid? It is certainly in every regulator's interest to make you think so. Insecure people mostly overcompensate and exaggerate in order to be heard. Our regulators are capable of both.

The case of Dr. Harold Shipman boosted the perceived need for medical regulators, even though they completely failed to detect him. Regulators will forever invoke him as an example of just how dangerous unregulated doctors can be, and how valuable regulators are to patient welfare.

Beware of Spies

Your colleagues, agencies such as the CQC, pharmacists, and the corporate bureaucrats you work with are the ones most likely to report any supposed infringement you make of '*Good Medical Practice*', NICE guidelines, or BNF directives. Any good you have done will not stand to your credit.

To have avoided patient complaints for over fifty years, while undertaking invasive cardiology and dealing with difficult to resolve medical cases (patients mostly came to me because other doctors had failed to help), is not an insignificant matter. In my dealings with the MPTS, GMC, and PSA., they gave no consideration to my record. This illustrates the sagacity of their actions, and stands as a measure of their blinkered assessments and judgements.

Towards the end of my career, dealing with anonymous, detached bureaucrats became tiresome and irrelevant. For junior doctors and nurses, the consequences of incurring regulatory proceedings can prove lifechanging. Regulators mean them to be. Having had a lifelong distrust of bureaucratic and corporate organisations, I never allowed my future to rest in their hands without some trepidation. I only worked a few years for the NHS. I appreciate that this is not a usual career path for most nurses and doctors in the UK, there being few alternative employers.

The only way out of the regulatory bind that the medical profession now finds itself in is to change the system. Medical regulators and their ever-growing bureaucratic legions enjoy power and considerable financial rewards, so they will strongly resist change. Because of my age, and strong disinclination to deal with any more corporate drones (a mutual feeling, no doubt), I will leave this mission to those of you with enough time, energy and political inclination for a fight.

Image Problems

Corporations are concerned about their image; some wish to hide from having one. When they failed to discover Dr. Harold Shipman, and the danger he presented to the public, the public image of medical regulators suffered. Where were they while he was killing hundreds of his patients? The GMC states on its website that: 'We work to protect patient safety and support medical education and practice across the UK.' The CQC states their mission to be: 'We make sure health and social care services provide people with safe, effective, compassionate, high-quality care and we encourage care services to improve.' I wonder if the families of Shipman's victims thought they did a good job.

Although they have no capacity to prevent harm to patients, medical regulators possess a perverse prophylactic power over healthcare workers. By inducing fear and trepidation, they make doctors and nurses think twice before engaging with patients and before taking any risk which might affect them. They did not induce fear and trepidation in Shipman. He was completely unconcerned about medical regulatory retribution. He killed his patients regardless. A junior employee at a local funeral director's office sealed his fate, not a medical regulator. She asked questions about his practice, one of which was 'why are so many of his patients dying?'

Allowing patients to die is easy; curing them and caring

for them requires a little more skill.

Many executives who work for faceless medical organisations prefer to remain anonymous. Their aim is to avoid personal responsibility and worry.

> *'In some respects, a society in which the members reach a universal level in which they are anonymous drones by choice is even more frightening than one in which they are forced to be so.'* — *John P. Getty (1986). How to be Rich. Penguin Publishing Group.*

Regulators and Errors of Judgment

Because of their background and education, we cannot expect medical regulators to respect the science of medicine or its practice, although nothing stops them from learning about it at an elementary level. The fixed laws they must use can mirror those of science, but can be incongruous when the real-time, fluid clinical judgements are made by doctors on behalf of patients. To help patients, doctors may have to depart from fixed rules and engage with the art of medicine in a responsive rather than in a fixed manner.

Do regulators know it is perfectly legitimate for scientists, physicians, and surgeons to have opposing views based on the same data? In choosing medical experts whose views support their case during MPTS trials, they strongly influence decisions in their favour. The same bias is open to the defence. If tribunal members understand nothing much about medical practice, except for general practice, what quality of justice can they mete out? If they protest, they will have only the weakest of lamentable defences like 'we did our best!' Can any society really afford to dispense with doctors based on the judgments of lawyers and laypeople with inadequate qualifications for judging them? The skills and education invested in every doctor are of immense value to every society, and not worth losing for wrong or trivial reasons. To achieve that, the value of regulators to society will need reassessment.

Guidelines used as Tramlines

I have mentioned this topic before, but it is important enough to expand on. Without a medical perspective, the GMC can ignore the fact that the BNF and NICE 'guidelines' need interpreting relative to clinical context. This results in them using guidelines as fixed rules, without deeming any discussion necessary (they are not qualified for either medical or scientific discussion). They simply want to use guidelines as legal instruments of compliance. Such misuse of guidelines does no justice to clinical medicine. The daily (sometimes hourly) variations in the clinical state of patients can make frequent reinterpretation of protocols and guidelines essential.

Here are a few observations about the application of fixed rules (tramlines) in medical practice:

1. No guideline will apply to every patient at all times. Patients are liable to suffer if we do not take their clinical circumstances into account (a point emphasised in all NICE guidelines). A guideline can be clinically inappropriate at one moment and completely appropriate at another. There is danger in thinking

that any guideline is immutable.

2. In every clinical forum where a patient's welfare is being discussed, we must always consider NICE guidelines. This is because NICE guidelines are based on evidence and balanced by experts in each field. Only detached, algorithmic thinkers will accept them unconditionally. Consideration of appropriateness is the prerogative of experienced clinicians, not lawyers. This is one means by which medical bureaucratic systems have achieved primacy over the medical profession.

3. Good medical practice must always include the art of medicine. Unfortunately for those lawyers, scientists, or businesspeople sitting in judgement on doctors and nurses, measuring it meaningfully (and reproducibly) is impossible.

These factors are all beyond the remit of current MPTS proceedings. Although vital to those accused, they will not be included in the legal consideration or considered in your defence. Such omissions represent social crimes against those who save lives and try their best to preserve the health of patients.

We must review the composition of MPTS tribunals. We should change their current composition to one composed only of senior doctors used to taking clinical risks, those who can interpret scientific evidence, and those who understand the art of practising medicine.

Disregard for the Statistical Paradox

Not only doctors abuse statistics. Most of those who call on statistics for evidence will quote a headline summary without looking for, or pointing to, the devils in the detail. At MPTS tribunals, and in doctors' consulting rooms, many will ignore the statistical paradox (that group data analysis cannot apply reliably to any individual), and favour the assumption of relevance. In applying most statistical results to individual patients, doctors must make their best guess. Although often expedient, this may involve erroneous extrapolation, inductive reasoning and guesswork. It is an art, not a science, to interpret research trial results and how they apply to specific patients.

Modus Operandi:
No Exceptions Allowed

At one MPTS Tribunal I attended, the barrister acting for the GMC refused to accept my description of two patients I had known for decades. They were a married couple, and 'exceptional' people. They were both exceptionally intelligent, exceptionally responsible, highly professional, and with jobs needing exceptional trust.

I trusted them to take 0.5mgs of lorazepam at night without dose escalation (I also trusted them to store fifty 1mg tablets, without fear of abuse). They had maintained unchanging doses for thirty years! Because of their high-ranking jobs in banking and the insurance industry, they were both trusted to manage high-value assets for others, so only the criminally minded would think them unexceptional. They both insisted that their medication improved their sleep and had no side-effects (repeated annual examinations and clinical investigations found no physical changes). I wanted them to give evidence, but my appointed barrister said it was pointless. They could add nothing to my case, and their views would be marked as hearsay.

Given that all patients differ from one another (except perhaps identical twins), an 'exceptional' state applies to all those who are not average (34% of cases in many 'normal' statistical distributions). The only way that doctors can deal with this individual variation is to assume reasonable similarity to the average. For any defined characteristic (sensitivity to pharmaceuticals, responsiveness of blood pressure, blood coagulability, and immune responses), most results fall within two standard deviations of the mean or mode of the population studied. This implies that our treatment policies and management will mostly apply to the majority. The key word here is 'mostly', but never 'always'.

One of these 'exceptional' patients of mine oversaw 25% of the branches of a major UK high street bank. Her husband (the other exceptional patient), worked at Lloyd's of London. Who would regard their levels of personal responsibility as 'average', I wonder? In deciding whether they were trustworthy and intelligent enough to take and keep a store of lorazepam, without escalating doses, the metainformation about their characters and roles was crucial to my therapeutic decisions. Unfortunately, members of an MPTS tribunal found this irrelevant. The BNF guideline to restrict benzodiazepine to short-term usage was relatively recent (the BNF committee found insufficient data to condone their long-term use). Both my patients had started on lorazepam a decade before anyone thought it wise to restrict it to the short-term.

I must emphasise that every experienced physician will know patients who could never be trusted to maintain the same dose of any drug, let alone an addictive one.

The suitability of patients to take responsibility and to act reliably, may have no quantitative measure, but they are qualities easily recognised by those experienced in life and business. With little or no care for pastoral involvement, and only a few minutes for each consultation, only a few detached NHS doctors actually consider them. Because I was in private practice, the involvement I had with my patients was different. I formed my judgement of the character of my two patients over several decades, having always spent thirty to sixty minutes in consultation with them each time we met. Lengthy personal engagement of this sort allows one to affirm important patient characteristics repeatedly. Since most doctors who work for the MPTS will be employed by the NHS, they will assume its sacred cow status despite the time restrictions and many other disadvantages the NHS imposes. MPTS tribunals are therefore unlikely to recognise the advantages patients have when they attend private practices like mine (another exception to the rule, I suspect).

Mutual evaluation is reliable only after a long and continuous exposure of a doctor to her patient. This is not now a feature of NHS practice, even though it is a prerequisite for practicing the art of medicine. The MPTS could not have understood my relationship with these patients, and might therefore have thought that I invented my patient's exceptional status. They therefore rejected the notion. Unwittingly comparing my practice to an NHS GPs practice was not comparing like with like. It resulted in a serious error of judgement on their part.

If the MPTS, GMC and CQC continue to deny that doctors are reliable judges of patients' characters, and are incapable of wise clinical judgement in individual cases, they will reduce doctors to processing patients algorithmically. All regulators will favour this. They can more easily control robots than doctors and nurses. Robots are unthinkingly compliant, and can apply blanket rules to every situation, regardless of any clinical common sense. It is regrettable that the intelligent, prudent, wise, independent-thinking medical profession I joined sixty years ago is now buried beneath pyramids of self-preserving bureaucrats using only rule books and algorithms. None I have ever met had any practical in-depth knowledge of how medical practice works, and how it can best serve patients.

Following the French Revolution, citizens were required to devote themselves to the First Republic of France. Those who wished to pursue a private life with independent ideas risked execution. 'The Revolution suffered citizens to live only as an expression, and servant of its interest. Life had legitimacy only when lived within the terms it dictated.' (*The Private Life*. Josh Cohen. Granta p39, 2013). The Bolsheviks had much the same idea. Are there similarities here to how our medical regulators wish to control the medical profession?

The medical profession as it now exists is one I was happy to quit. My resignation from the medical profession in the UK became obligatory for me, given the many objections I held (and still hold) about the way doctors and nurses are treated, regulated, and policed. To be consistent in my derogation of medical corporations imposing senseless rules, I also resigned my membership of the RCP, and the RSM (although I never knew either professional body to act senselessly. I was always proud to belong to both). My resignation removed any obligation they might have had to me.

My most happy resignation was from the CQC. This was after they decided I had become an unsuitable provider (to direct a clinic in which other doctors might work). None of my patients agreed with them. No doctor I knew agreed with them. So are patients really their concern? Since every corporation is but a convenient business structure staffed by anonymous bureaucrats, it cannot be capable of concern. It is interesting to note just how many corporations, try to express false ideas of concern. Many train their receptionists to say 'have a nice day', but how often is this another insincere corporate wish?

During my MPTS appearances, never did they seek to assess my clinical acumen, experience, style of practice, success in handling risk, or the characteristics of my patients (socioeconomic background, employment, education, responsibilities, and job details). It was clearly irrelevant to their algorithmic decision-making processes.

It soon became clear to me that the MPTS tribunal and I were singing from different hymn sheets. They were using one finger to play 'Do-Re-Mi' in C major (the least complicated of keys to play on a piano); my scores were all written for a whole orchestra to play in D minor!

At the end of the last day of my MPTS tribunal hearing, I told them what I thought of their medicolegal processes (in a letter delivered by my barrister. See Appendix 1). I did not return the following morning for their verdict (one year suspension). I regarded them as unfit to judge any doctor or their medical practice without respecting all the crucial metainformation. They were not going to agree with my dissent, so why would I bother to reappear for sentencing the next day?

Should the MPTS ever ignore the learning, individual experience, and reasoned intellectual standpoint of any doctor in matters involving clinical management? They may have this right in law, but that does not make what they decide sensible, wise or clinically correct. Their decisions will not be just while they persist in ignoring the reality of dealing with patients.

Shock and Awe

Fear of medical regulators is now profound among many members of the medical profession in the UK. Doctors and nurses will need more than malpractice insurance to defend themselves in court. Some will need counselling. Like all other penal organisations, medical regulators can presume that all the allegations they make are true until proven otherwise. What may follow can be a protracted legal process. The stress and anguish caused will diminish the work performance of many accused. Because the process is protracted, outsiders will get the impression that the GMC tries to deal with cases considerately and in a just way. The protracted period is caused by their inefficiency, not by their considerateness. At least the delays can allow an accused doctor to continue her valuable work, albeit with a Damoclean sword hanging over her head.

The GMC is the most feared of medical regulators, but the CQC also enjoys the statutory right to induce dismay, shock and awe in doctors, nurses, and practice managers. They have methods to keep it so, but then their job is important, making sure that patients receive a certain minimum standard of in-house service. Effective housekeeping functions are rightly their concern, as are the nature of the services offered by every practice. If doctors and their practices are fully compliant, they have nothing to fear. In order to achieve that, time and money will have to be spent that might better be spent directly on patients.

CQC inspectors can visit unannounced (although not usually), sanction spies (outside stakeholders) to investigate practices, and make public their judgements of doctors and their practices. Their views and reports rest on pre-set, tick-box, binary criteria, regardless of clinical pertinence. They need not officially include the views of the doctors they visit, but they should. CQC inspectors cannot entertain clinical or academic discussion, although they might engage in judging clinical issues if one of their inspectors is medically qualified.

Doctors and nurses must never forget that dealing with any regulator is a legal encounter, not a clinical one. It is essential to have witnesses and to record everything that is said as evidence. Better still, the proceedings should be recorded. Doctors who fight fire with fire might gain the respect of some inspectors. It might dent their sanctimony, but don't rely on it.

Like the GMC, the CQC can choose to ignore the fact that most experienced doctors are educated, sentient beings with valuable academic and practical points of view to express. These are not the characteristics of too many corporate employees. Doctors and nurses all have views that regulatory corporations could learn. Unfortunately learning is not their brief. Inspectors are corporate representatives positioned well outside the realities of medical practice. Inspectors will listen, but only because they have been trained to. They rely on scripted questions and replies, agreed beforehand at HQ. Their legal mission is simple: collect as much evidence as possible. Compliance with their rules and regulations is their only concern. They will try not to waste time on anything else, but will be completely unconcerned about the time doctors and nurses will lose for dealing with patients.

I once challenged CQC inspectors with the fact that I had practiced privately at the Loughton Clinic for over forty-seven years without a single patient complaining of being mismanaged. My rhetorical question was: how is it that the CQC is not interested in learning how I achieved this? Their visits are scripted, with no need to learn anything from any doctor. I have sometimes enjoyed wasting my time challenging bureaucrats; it relieves boredom and reflects my sardonic East London sense of humour. Anybody who holds the view that rules set in stone are the best way to govern any professional practice, be it clinical medicine or otherwise, is a fool not worthy of your time. Dealing with the CQC is a job for managers with corporate sympathies, not for medical professionals.

> *There is nothing new about the unchanging problem of power, and its application: it is 'often abused once acquired'. —Alexander Hamilton (1757-1804).*
> *'It is hard to imagine a more stupid or more dangerous way of making decisions than by putting (those) decisions in the hands of people who pay no price for being wrong.'*
> — *Thomas Sowell.*

With some bravado born of their statutory authority (CQC inspectors will brandish their badges of authority if you question it), CQC inspectors now assume they appreciate doctor patient relationships and the work doctors do. They cannot, of course, but their statutory authority gives them the right to harbour the delusion. Medical regulators have come to harbour a more serious delusion. They think that their authority allows them to exceed the medical sovereignty gifted to doctors by their patients (based on medical knowledge, ability, and experience, sufficient to save and improve their lives). While medical regulatory bureaucrats can claim to act in the public interest, and guard the safety of the public from potentially dangerous medical professionals, it is doctors and nurses who hold the trust of millions.

The CQC has some valuable functions: maintaining minimal standards of cleanliness, inspecting building safety, and assuring the safety of the equipment used. Instead of limiting themselves to these housekeeping functions for which they are undoubtedly qualified, they are now poised to expand their powers. Common to every CQC inspection was something I found rather worrying. Inspectors (even medically qualified ones) clearly undervalue the clinical judgement and experience of doctors.

For the first few decades of my professional life, I was completely unaware of bureaucratic involvement. With or without them, doctors and nurses were always ready to step forward and help patients. There are now many doctors and nurses so in fear of being accused of noncompliance, they must consider letting a patient die in front of them. Perhaps that's not so bad! Regulatory bureaucrats will commend them for their excellent compliance with regulations.

Medical Tribunals v Legal Tribunals

Lawyers can function in a medical arena by restricting themselves to compliance issues, and by falsely accepting guidelines as immutable rules. The regulatory system has a staffing problem. If only highly qualified senior GPs, medical academics, consultant physicians and surgeons are expert enough to decide the value of the guidelines in each case, what might induce them to do this sort of work?

The GMC has an appropriate purpose, given its legal staffing structure. That is to establish criminal behaviour. Instead they also bring serious consequences to competent doctors, too easily sanctioned for matters which most practising clinicians would regard as minor or fatuous. Somehow the GMC as a legal corporation has been tasked to represent the clinical interests of both patients and the medical profession. These matters need a public airing as a prequel to necessary organisational changes. Changing a corporation full of anonymous operatives, hiding from public scrutiny, will be a challenge. We need to question their fitness to 'safeguard the public, and the public interest'. We must also question their fitness to 'safeguard the public from doctors and nurses, and . . . to protect the reputation of the medical profession'.

David Dighton

Regulatory Reform: The Need for a Medical Directorate

Medical regulatory agencies as they are now composed (legally based, supported mostly by third-party NHS doctors, with financial reasons for allegiance) cannot hope to appreciate how each medical practice functions at street level. Their lack of appreciation or acceptance, of all that I have considered here, makes their judgement of clinical matters unsafe. Only doctors with sufficient pertinent clinical experience, openly prepared to discuss the medical technical aspects and metadata of each case, can hope to judge the clinical validity of allegations made against doctors. Clinical allegations against doctors and nurses will have a technical context that will vary from case to case. Only those who understand clinical context will appreciate it. For this reason alone, legally oriented regulatory bodies should become involved only after patients have been harmed, have complained of harm, or have died.

If any doctor should claim an appreciation of the workings of the law without the education and experience necessary, would they not deserve mockery? Medical regulators in the same position, however, dare to claim an understanding of medical practice. But that is to miss the point. Their job is simply to decide whether a law or a guideline has been breached. They need not pretend to have any clinical understanding. They will claim to use third-party, medically trained expert advisers with clinical expertise, for that. Both can give rise to errors in a system claiming to judge the work of nurses and doctors fairly.

It would require a completely independent medical

directorate to get judgements of doctors and nurses that include an experienced clinical perspective. It would require the involvement of all the Royal Colleges. Only they could approve doctors with the most pertinent experience. On occasions it would be appropriate for those offering clinical judgement to have visited the doctor and his practice. They could then question all involved, and see the doctor and his practice at first hand, not at third hand. This is a minimum requirement for insightful assessment given the contributions doctors make to society.

GMC lawyers should only become involved when harm to a patient is alleged, or there is undeniable evidence of criminality. In such cases, a medical tribunal's duties would be to refer the accused to the most appropriate legal agency (the MPTS, or courts of law). The GMC's role would be to ratify the judgements of medical tribunals. Decisions of the MPTS are now protected from GMC interference, and the Medical Directorate I propose would need the same protection from the GMC and PSA.

Only a medical directorate tribunal would have enough expertise and experience to discuss a doctor's past and future clinical risk taking, and any need for further training. Learning, not vengeance, needs to set the direction of travel. We should allow a medical directorate to recommend a change in regulations and guidelines, especially when a doctor on trial has given nothing but benefit to his patients. Funding for further research could also be part of their remit.

The GMC will object to all such changes. They will remind us of their statutory powers. They will argue that medical self-regulation is dangerous, an example of anti-democratic nepotism and cronyism. They will doubtless argue that it is neither in the public interest nor in the interest of the medical profession.

In order to safeguard 'public interest', every medical tribunal should have a duty to listen to the patients of accused doctors and take their comments into account. Their testimony needs to be given due respect and weight, and not simply rejected as hearsay. They are voters and not unimportant. When a doctor is being judged by outsiders a quorum of the most important people involved, the doctor's patients, should be co-opted to give evidence. Some will have entrusted their lives to the doctor on trial and will have valuable contributions to make.

In order to assess the risk a doctor might present in the future, the MPTS insists on witnessing his remorse, contrition and a willingness to learn (in ways they will find acceptable). To be seen in a favourable light, barristers will direct their clients to show obsequious respect for the process, and to demonstrate a strong intent to comply in the future. This is all easily feigned. In my case, knowing that the MPTS had appreciated none of my clinical and individual practice factors, neither contrition nor a desire to learn from my mistakes was appropriate. With all my patients happy with my management, and no harm done to any of them over many decades, any remorse I showed would have been disingenuous.

There was always one elephant in the MPTS tribunal rooms I attended. My not complying fully with the demands of a regulator, and not showing them the respect they thought they deserved, were the tacit crucial issues (my solicitor had previously described my initial responses to GMC allegations as 'robust'). Obviously I lacked sufficient insight and respect for their awesome power and authority. Having experienced their lack of understanding of me, my practice, and my patients, what other position could I hold honourably? Because my contempt for them occurred simultaneously with my desire to retire, I had no need to play Sisyphus and respect their weighty boulder of authority. No large boulder, or any legal corporation I know, can claim clinical sensibility and wisdom.

Medical practice was my life for over sixty years after entering medical school. During that time, I experienced all the good that medical practice can bring to patients. Why then, should any doctor have to feign respect for regulators when they can so easily disregard doctors and the medical profession in their legal proceedings? This is a cultural issue. The culture expressed by the GMC and MPTS is that the sanctity of the law is above the need for medical practice. For me, no man-made law deserves primacy over saving lives and the relief of suffering.

I fully appreciate that few doctors will be able to follow my lead in relation to regulators. I hope, at least, that knowing the facts of my case will sharpen their attitudes towards them, help them change the system, and keep them in their rightful subordinate place. I will never accept that those who work for legal corporations can compete in value with those who save lives and reduce suffering in a society. I humbly agree with Socrates. He thought it right to suggest the division of people (and professions) into different value groups.

The future of medicine lies in the hands of doctors and nurses with enough honest ability and knowledge to bring about improvements in patient morbidity and mortality. The satisfaction patients get from the medical services they pay for is important. We should not allow doctors to be suspended or removed from the medical register simply because they have not complied with a questionable regulatory rule, or a bureaucratic guideline, not without academic medical discussion, and the review of experienced clinical experts who will know how to take all the metainformation into account.

Retribution

The GMC and CQC have been successful in providing deterrents, but do they really believe their actions remove only substandard doctors, lessen future clinical risk, and improve patient safety?

Any system based on blame, retribution, and absolute compliance, with a culture dedicated to punishment rather than learning, will seek scapegoats. Because doctors are clever and used to learning, scapegoat status is both disrespectful and inappropriate. Medicine must strive to leave negativity behind and emulate the airline industry. Let's analyse every fault, catastrophe, and near catastrophe like they do so that we can all learn and progress safely. We will achieve this by disseminating all we have learned from accidents and mishaps. The appraisal of every doctor should include a measure of such learning (as it does for pilots).

At the moment medical regulators (very few of whom are doctors), are paid to pursue us, and to dispense retribution and public vengeance without getting specific permission from the public. Patients give their indirect permission by voting for politicians, twenty times removed from their medical and personal issues. Their primary purpose should not be to uncover culprits and dissenters, and punish them in the name of public safety. This culture is wrong. We should recast the laws to respect the fact that few pilots get up in the morning wishing to crash into a mountain, and very few doctors and nurses awake wishing to harm their patients.

Nick Ross, during an RSM webinar ('When things go wrong. Doctors in the dock'), made several important points about the retribution and vengeance delivered by legal processes in the name of justice. Shaming, blaming and punishing in order to exact vengeance do not deter crime, reduce the occurrence of accidents, or reduce noncompliance, as many believe. Yet opinion remains polarised.

There are those who believe that we need more punishment in order to deter crime, and those who believe that understanding and education will work better. Despite public hangings (stopped in the UK in 1868), crime remained rife. If shaming and blaming worked, there would be fewer than six million in the UK still smoking, fewer ignoring the problems of obesity, many more wearing safety belts, and fewer talking on their mobile phones while driving.

In the eyes of medical bureaucrats, few make better scapegoats than principled, dedicated doctors and nurses; some of whom have records showing decades of beneficial service to patients and no harm.

Just to remind you, in this book, I have not been discussing the fifteenth century Spanish Inquisition. My subject has been medical regulators in control of the plight of UK doctors, nurses, and other healthcare workers in 2023. With an increasing number of UK doctors and nurses choosing to retrain, or go elsewhere, their control needs urgent review.

Chapter 3:
Future Medical Practice

There are two technical innovations about to revolutionise medical practice: the use of genetic profiling, and expert AI systems (what the NHS calls 'Digital First').

The corporate structure and ethos of the NHS has caused many inadequacies that cannot remain hidden. As a dysfunctional system, it deprives many UK patients of the care they deserve.

There are two management system changes needed to improve the regulation of UK medical practice:

1. The creation of a Medical Directorate advised by the Royal Colleges with statutory authority equal to but independent of the GMC and the Public Services Authority. A Medical Directorate responsible for the conduct of the medical profession, in all clinical matters.

2. A change in NHS bureaucratic culture, from primarily preserving the NHS and its corporate ethos to primarily preserving patients by once again recognising the work of medical professionals as sacrosanct.

While the management of the NHS continues to use corporate principles detached from medical experience and knowhow, a clinically guided medical service for patients will remain a fantasy. Only older patients will know what we have lost from the NHS over the decades. A few in their late eighties and nineties might remember medicine as it was before the NHS. Some will remember a time when they had their own GP, one they could easily contact, and who knew them and their family personally (and sometimes four generations of the same family). They will remember doctors providing pastoral care and the considerate availability of help in casualty and cottage hospitals. They will remember convalescent homes, and self-motivated nurses and doctors dedicated to their work and driven by a strong vocation.

The continuity, availability, and pastoral care GPs once offered five decades ago should be restored as the only basis for a medical service that will satisfy patient's medical needs to the full. GPs once each managed 3000 patients. Today some GPs complain about having 1000 patients on their list!

> *Relabelling is one way to achieve the impression of corporate progress. Since before Hippocrates, doctors have advised patients about their diet, exercise, and other lifestyle issues as part of pastoral care. By relabelling this as 'social prescribing', bureaucracy can now claim progress over what went before.*

NHS medical practice functions in a culturally distinct way from independent private practice. As a result they each have different patient outcomes. Equivalent differences in efficiency and effectiveness exist between every nationalised industry and private enterprise. Both can learn something useful from the other.

Is it time to separate the control and supervision of these two medical cultures: the NHS and private practice? Should we promote private medical schools, and nurture the ethos that has forever embraced the more personal type of medicine found in our private sector? Because the cultural divide between the two remains deep, those who inspect practices and regulate doctors should know and respect the differences. As it is at the moment, they are so different, they should be regulated differently. One might suggest that the most acceptable features of each are adopted by both, although it will meet resistance from the deeply imbedded culture of the NHS. Most UK medical professionals are totally invested in NHS practice culture, and will see no need to change, even if patients might prefer it.

Over the last decade, I have noticed some changes in both systems. Private hospitals were once like five-star hotels, clearly valuing their customers from the moment they appeared (since customers are all free to choose from many other good hotels). As private hospitals have taken on NHS patients, their approach has become more dismissive (patients are not all like they used to be). Their receptionists are now much more likely to give their computer screen priority than the patient standing before them. NHS practices now seem more accommodating, with less fire-breathing and dismissiveness on display.

Both NHS and private practice have much to learn from one another, but with the unresolved, shocking health divide that the government and the NHS preside over, it will be our national service that needs to learn most. Private practice has the easy job, traditionally presiding over the rich with their lower morbidity and mortality from whatever medical condition they endure. Can we transplant any of its patient-centred ethos into the corporate NHS machine? As I said before, I sometimes enjoy asking pointless, rhetorical questions!

What Defines the Medical Service Cultural Divide?

From all I have seen, NHS doctors and nurses value their patients the same as private doctors and nurses, but the character of each service is different. In private practice, patients are treated like clients staying in expensive hotels; their custom is valued. The same contrast exists between supermarkets and small, proprietor-run businesses. Supermarkets can enjoy anonymity, but will help if asked; small shops mostly take pride in personal service and developing a relationship with each customer. Corporations are rule-based and need to develop a standardised approach; small businesses and private doctors can personalise their approach to each customer and patient. For these reasons it is practicable to regard the NHS and private practice as having different cultures. They must therefore be regulated and judged differently.

Private practice culture means that all patients can expect to discuss their medical matters (on the telephone or otherwise) directly with the doctor of their choice. Same-day appointments are usual for private GP patients. Investigation results are available within twenty-four hours, and consultant appointments are available quickly, with less need for consulting time restriction. All these exist in the NHS, but are rarer. There are no private hospital waiting lists to speak of, and quicker patient turnarounds. Because private patients are richer than average (or have been up until recently), private patient outcomes have always been on the safer side of the national health divide, with the best of patient morbidity and mortality.

Patient management is a main feature of the cultural difference. In the NHS, management bureaucrats have a status above that of doctors and nurses, and their salaries and authority reflect it. NHS inertia is caused (like all nationalised industries) by a surfeit of governing bodies, decision-making committees, government fiscal restrictions (by those with legal and business degrees, not medical degrees), too many managers (with no clinical perspective), and too few staff doing the work of caring. There are too many organisational knots and logjams, too much functional red tape leading to poor integration of services, inefficiency in patient handling, and too many corporate requirements for audit and feedback with no motivation to change, even in the face of patient dissatisfaction and mounting lawsuits. The NHS is too big to fail, and, as a sacred cow that is part of our British identity, too respected to admit the many faults patients now level at it. The system is not about to be unravelled, so only revolutionary change will improve it.

Health Maintenance Organisations (HMOs): Are they the way forward?

In the USA, Health Maintenance Organisations (HMOs) accept monthly pre-payments for medical services provided to patients under contract. Pre-payment, whether in hotels (all-inclusive deals), or medical facilities, will affect the attitude of both staff and customers (patients) in definable ways. Staff can become de-personalised. HMO staff know that the patients have rights, subject to contract. Patients know exactly what they have paid for, and will insist on getting it. The disputes that arise can detract from the doctor patient relationship. HMO schemes could be more acceptable to the British public than a recent suggestion for every NHS hospital inpatient to pay £8 to £10 per day.

One supreme motivating force in the private medical sector is creating profit. Financial matters must never concern medical staff, whether in the NHS, or the private sector. The care of patients is too important for that. Their concern should always be patient welfare, regardless of cost. Unfortunately, in the private sector, self-paying patients and the reluctance of private insurance companies to pay can sometimes limit the clinical possibilities.

David Dighton

Medicine and Artificial Intelligence

Expert computer systems rather than AI, have already provided helpful apps for patients, and many more for nurses and doctors. Despite the dismay voiced by the RCGP and by GPs who are losing their patients (and their NHS capitation fees) to online doctors, convenience will ensure further progress in this direction.

In all business sectors providing convenience has become essential to commercial success. Opportunistic, online doctors will solve a major problem for NHS patients: availability. They will eventually provide the convenience of twenty-four-hour consultation services linked to twenty-four-hour pharmacy delivery services.

Do we still need to examine patients? The current fashion for telemedicine excludes the possibility, except for picturing physical signs in photos and videos. One can visualise skin conditions, cyanosis, jaundice, ankle oedema and even a raised JVP, although setting the camera at the right angle in indirect light would be difficult to achieve. A significant minority of tele-consultations must end with the same advice: 'go and see your doctor!'

Nurses trained to use diagnostic apps will undoubtedly take over more and more functions from GPs. If I were a young GP today, I would plan my retreat into another area of work, or aim to be a consultant GP, supervising a team of nurses, paramedics, pharmacists and other ancillary medical workers.

NHS accountants will have already calculated the money to be saved by replacing doctors with

AI. They will hardly object to GPs losing patients to private systems like the Babylon-based digital practice in Fulham, West London. It will reduce NHS GP workload. The once Minister for Health, Matt Hancock, joined it in 2018, as have over 30,000 others. This move will mean the loss of capitation fees for NHS GPs.

Nurses already undertake several specialised clinics in the UK, NHS general practices. Since they are adept at following rules and guidelines (more than free-thinking doctors), they will readily deliver a CQC approved, rule-based service for patients. A future practice might comprise two consultant GPs and ten nurses, with paramedics and physiotherapists who can handle chronic rheumatic cases (20% of all patients seen). The current argument is that GPs are irreplaceable, and we need many more of them. If this plan does not lead to improved public convenience, it will not happen. So far, GPs have not proven themselves to be available as much as the public would like. Parkinson's Law predicts that more of them will do little to improve their efficiency.

Paramedical Medicine

In comparison with NHS GPs, practice nurses and pharmacists are likely to provide better continuity. Since most UK patients have little technical knowledge of medicine, someone less qualified, like a nurse, pharmacist, or paramedic, could easily become a preferred provider if more conveniently available. In my early days most patients consulted their GPs for a certificate of some sort, or a repeat prescription. Someone other than a doctor could easily provide such services (with back-up available). Nurses handle a lot of medical management as it is (asthma, diabetes, hypertension), so why not extend their remit? For many paramedics, nurses and pharmacists, the possibility of taking on further clinical roles must be exciting. Doctors would then also have an opportunity. They could engage with in-depth medicine and the more challenging demands of hospital medicine and surgery. The future role of doctors would be made more technical, and distinct from the roles played by nurses, paramedics, and pharmacists.

Future Algorithms and Common Sense

It is important to know that a doctor's career may soon lie in the hands of algorithmic thinkers, bureaucrats conceited enough to think that with medical AI, they can legitimately wield clinical power over doctors and nurses. My medical education never prepared me for dealing with the hollow men of bureaucracy, but this is now an essential skill. The NHS, CQC, GMC, and PSA rely on algorithmic functioning. This reflects their regulatory, rule-based culture. Since they will doubtless expand their use of apps in the future, the medical profession must give thought to all the implications.

The best character judgements of others can be made when trivial matters are observed. Here is one trivial example of what the algorithmic thinking of the GMC can do:

The GMC told Dr. P.M., a young doctor that she needed to take an English language test if she wanted to work in the UK. She was born in a foreign land, Australia, and qualified as a doctor in Australia. Her mother tongue is English, and nobody has ever called upon her to speak any other language. So why a language test? The answer lies in a faulty algorithmic process that cannot distinguish 'foreign doctors' from non-English-speaking countries from 'foreign doctors' coming from countries where English is the first language. An average eight-year-old would know the difference, but not the GMC!

Although this case defies common sense, it illustrates an emerging theme: the use of algorithmic thinking, accepted and applied without further thought. If you have just started your medical career, you will need to know that your career may no longer depend on the wise judgements of experienced senior clinicians. Love may or may not be blind, but linear algorithms always are.

We write algorithms as programming sequences to accept, process, and store data. Calculations like BMI and QRisk3 can then be made easily. Deciding which calculation is the most appropriate may rest on a simple rule of thumb. Sometimes calculations are made using a mathematical model, like the one initially used to estimate likely COVID-19 deaths in 2020. What will usually remain hidden and accepted without further thought are the mathematical formulae used, and the logical integrity of the programming.

On March 16th 2020, a twenty-page report on COVID-19 from Imperial College, London, estimated 510,000 deaths in the UK as a worst-case outcome: (a) if nothing were to be done in response to the COVID-19 pandemic, and (b) should an estimated reproduction number (r-rate) of 2.4 be correct. The estimate, resulting from a mathematical model (algorithmic calculation), proved to be an erroneous overestimate. (Reynolds, Alan. 2020.)

Models are always wrong, but some are useful
—George E. P. Box, FRS: Statistician.

Everyday happenings occur with familiar frequency. Typically they occur *'sometimes, but not always'* or *'rarely, but they will happen'*. The incidences that are not 'usual' will be underrepresented in every averaged statistical model (based on a Poisson distribution). Unusual occurrences are proverbial 'spanners in the works' for algorithms. The next big computing hope neural networks (programming systems that appear to learn, and update themselves with feedback) might 'learn' to handle exceptions, or at least come to know when they are out of their depth. Using all the same sort of considerations, would it also be reasonable to expect pigs to fly?

For human decision making and judgement to stand the test of time and prove wise, both must involve consideration of all the facts and metafacts, weighing each for relevance and giving each of them an appropriate priority. This is the basic requirement for all applicable clinical decisions. No fixed algorithm can balance relevance (they are omnivores, simply devouring whatever we feed them). One implication is vital to understand: their output will not always be correct.

The larger the organisation, the more it will rely on algorithmic thinking. Most large, successful corporations are algorithm-driven. Their fixed processes, and their size, both predict inertia. Resisting changes to their *modus operandi* is an inherent characteristic. Why change a formula that works, even if it ignores all individual considerations? Some people on a mission to change society, government thinking, or public attitudes will spend their lives battling with institutional inertia. So, is there an alternative?

I understand that in Silicon Valley, California, employees in some tech companies have the freedom to think freely and employ 'blue-sky thinking'. Free of regulated activity, they run profitable companies. There is a reason for this. Their atypical employees are intelligent and insightful enough for self-regulation. Those with less ability need to follow algorithmically- driven directives. The 'blue-sky thinking' model works only with highly intelligent, self-motivated people. This is not a practicable universal alternative to the algorithmic management culture, but one that can run in parallel.

Digital machines function with easily distributed programs (algorithms). Those who wish to control the practice of medicine with algorithms have a major problem: medicine does not function in a predictable, controlled manner. Unlike digitally controlled machines, serendipity and unpredictability are part of everyday life for doctors and nurses. Because computer programming literacy is uncommon, computer science will easily bemuse those who know little about it. Many of them populate the halls of medical bureaucracy and regulation, with many biased in favour of what they cannot understand. The biases involved are the incomprehensible bias, the framing bias, the automation bias, the bandwagon bias, the information bias, and the Travis effect bias.

We can expect regulators to be eager about the advantages of the digital revolution, with its potential for control. To enforce their rules easily, they only need to apply a rigid preprogrammed algorithmic system for regulating the standards of medical practice. This has metaphorical equivalents: allowing kindergarten children to write the rules, not their teachers, and to allow passengers to fly aeroplanes instead of trained pilots.

As the public becomes more dependent on phone apps, the judgements of experienced, knowledgeable people will become downrated in value by most people, but not by those who know the value of knowledge and experience.

Captivated by mobile telephone and computer screens, few realise what data those who direct and control their communication systems can capture. Although many acknowledge that surreptitious collection data is ubiquitous, most of us ignore it.

Some Basic Medical Practice Objectives

Every doctor and nurse should aim to achieve (or retrieve) the following objectives, none of which have changed for millennia:

1. To put our patient's welfare before our own.
2. Be knowledgeable and effective, successful enough medically to gain the trust of patients.
3. Be worthy of a sovereign medical duty: doctors taking primary responsibility for the life and death of their patients (should they request or need it).
4. Act as the director, producer, and coordinator of all that is necessary to manage patient health and illness.
5. Become efficient enough to bring the best diagnostic and clinical management skills to bear for each patient

in the shortest time possible.

6. Know each patient well enough to act as their advocate, especially when they have to deal with the advice of others, or a system not fit to foster their progress.

7. Act as the patient's defender and protagonist, safeguarding them from those who would interfere with their wishes, or transgress any doctor patient relationships they have developed.

8. Guard every patient's medical confidentiality.

As an illustration of the cultural differences, objectives 4 to 8 are much easier to attain in private practice than in NHS practice.

Putting Patients First

Sadly, this is no longer obligatory, but it should be! If doctors put their patients first, and it contravenes the GMC's '*Good Medical Practice*', they will risk punitive consequences. I was subject to these consequences, despite my patients being those others found difficult to diagnose and treat, and some of whom they had rejected (in order to keep their head below the bureaucratic parapet). This required my adherence to three principles:

1. The clinical buck stopped with me.

2. My patient's medical welfare always came first.

3. I tried my best for each patient, even if it risked harm (only with their fully informed consent), or risked regulatory retribution.

I always tried to adhere to all three. They served my patients well for five decades. In my case with the GMC, clause (2) served my patients well, but not me. Some say that medicine is a self-sacrificial profession. I continue to applaud the fact, even after becoming its victim (but not its martyr).

The buck should only stop with those who can claim sufficient expertise (in my case, the GMC correctly claimed that there were doctors more expert than I was in prescribing controlled drugs for addicts). In my case I could not find such a doctor for my patient, one who was acceptable to both me and my patient. This is a private practice problem, and not one that exists in the NHS. The patient duped me and did everything she could to avoid doctors who might have taken a stricter approach than me. I suspected this, and contacted some local pharmacists and her GP. Her GP then retired and my messages became lost to those who replaced him. This is an old story of little relevance, other than the warning it can provide for others.

Basic Objectives for Nurses

They should aim to:
1. Become effective enough to gain the trust of their patients.
2. To manage patients back to health with their nursing expertise, kindness, and any empathetic support they need.
3. Openly act as the patient's advocate, especially when they are not happy with the advice given by doctors and other professionals. This follows the path laid down by Florence Nightingale. Without her challenging those in charge, many more soldiers would have died in the

Crimean campaign (1853 to 1856).

Nurses to 'Bring Back Compassion!'

From the NHS ivory tower of reinventions, executive UK nurses published their undeniably excellent 'six C's' guidance for nursing care in 2012. They obviously thought that nurses and student nurses needed instruction in (or reminding of) the basic requirements for all nursing practice. The six C's are: care, compassion, courage, communication, commitment, and competence. One motive must have been to make Florence Nightingale turn in her grave! After all, she had already established the same 'C's' by 1858 (see 'Notes on matters affecting the Health, Efficiency and Hospital Administration of the British Army').

Apart from the best, not every nurse I ever met excelled in each of the six C's. A few less dedicated nurses, primarily motivated by earning money, could have ignored them all. Times have changed. Are the six C's not now basic to every nurse's training, with only some needing to be reminded of them? Could it be that the NHS has tried to function without them (they are all time-consuming), but failed? Was it that the medically detached, ill-educated directors of the NHS were out of touch with medical reality, and had enough time on their hands to revivify old nursing values? These are values without which no nurse can be called a nurse. Perhaps they came to know, through audit and feedback, that a growing lack of compassion and care was tarnishing the NHS's nursing reputation? Perhaps we should congratulate them for trying to counter the trend while admitting their corporate failings?

Admissions of bureaucratic defeat are rare, and occur mostly when defeat is inevitable. The future will hopefully witness more of the same, because from the perspective of any experienced nurse or doctor, we need a lot more of the same. The need to restate the historic common sense and wisdom of Florence Nightingale was sad. It was perhaps a measure of NHS corporate nursing management, and a reflection of how the work of nurses is now regarded.

For yet another example of corporate BLindingly OBvious (BLOB), barn-door thinking, consider what came forth from the Academy of Medical Sciences (December 15th, 2015). They declared that health maintenance was better than disease orientation, and . . . wait for it . . . that 'prevention is better than cure'. They concluded that this was not arguable. Really! Both Hippocrates and Florence Nightingale will have turned in their graves.

These statements were doubtless the result of endless conference meetings, staffed by non-scientists, commissioned to understand what medicine is about and how it works. Why waste money, staff and resources? They could have saved time and asked those who already know what it is all about and how it works.

The Good Old Days

If you want to know the future, look at the past.
— Albert Einstein

My motivation for writing this book sprang from both sadness and nostalgia. The medical profession I joined as an eighteen-year-old medical student in 1961, at the London Hospital Medical School in London has changed somewhat.

I was only one of two non-public school boys admitted to my year. I was also one of a small minority who had not followed a parent into the medical profession. One factor aided my acceptance: I had passed eleven O-Level exams (GCSEs now) without having studied science at school. I was self-taught. This was something the dean, Dr. John Ellis, recognised as an important qualification. He thought doctors needed initiative to practise medicine. A willingness to comply with corporate rules and regulations has now replaced this selection criterion.

Few of the student nurses I encountered as a student needed to work. They mostly came from privileged, wealthy backgrounds, and nursing was their vocation.

When I entered medical school, the Second World War had been over only sixteen years. That meant my teachers (most of whom had served in the armed forces) had little regard for long hours of work and tiredness. Once I qualified, nobody discussed hours of work or pay.

The hours of work now allowed for doctors and nurses may have changed, but their sense of duty and commitment to patients has not. The COVID-19 pandemic proved that. Most who work as medical professionals have altruistic sentiments and a commitment to duty, rarely found in other walks of life. But then we have our sovereign duties to perform. To be there for our patients, and to help them in every way we can, whatever it takes, and however long it takes. HM Queen Elizabeth awarded the George Cross to the NHS. The award recognised the 'courage, compassion and dedication' of NHS staff during the pandemic. In the early decades of my career, an NHS medical job did not attract a good salary. This made the altruistic more recognisable. Many junior doctors supplemented their income with locum work.

Most of my teachers were gentlemen and men of privilege. Some wore stiff collars, monocles, pince-nez, and pinstriped trousers (one wore tails). Although they were mostly formal, their modesty and lack of pretentiousness saw them treat dustmen (refuse collectors), and duchesses the same. Their behaviour portrayed 'good manners and behaviour' (the behaviour which leaves others feeling comfortable). I regret to say that their dignity, humility, and gentlemanly behaviour may have disappeared somewhat. The future is unlikely to see such formal behaviour return, with patients now preferring a more relaxed professional style.

For the sake of balance, let me counter my nostalgic idolatry with a negative anecdote. I was told by an anatomy demonstrator that I could not enter the medical school library on a Saturday morning without a jacket and tie! His intention was to enforce discipline and uphold dresscode standards.

As Yuval Noah Harari has it *('Sapiens: A Brief History of Humankind.* Vintage 2011*),* many institutions have a mythical image. The medical profession has always held an element of mystique, made all the more intriguing by special knowledge and capability, professional behaviour and formal attire. Is it a myth that the average doctor is better educated than the average person and has higher ethical standards than most? Is it a myth that Army officers differ from their men, or that state school pupils differ from their public-school contemporaries? Is it a myth that these are no longer important issues to those who choose medicine as a career?

No animal survives unless its behaviour fulfils an evolutionary purpose. The respectful formality of doctors helped maintain the trust and acceptance of patients. In the future, it may be positive work audits that count most.

When I was a junior doctor, no nonmedical person would have dared interfere in any doctor patient relationship. Decades before any need for accreditation and certification, the assumption was that doctors and nurses alone knew what was best for patients. Nurses, and never managers, facilitated the interventions doctors deemed necessary. Accountants, managers, and regulators were notable by their absence. They had no place in medical management or decision making. Closeted away somewhere, they concerned themselves with undoubtedly important practical tasks, like keeping the hospital functioning, staffing, provisioning, cleaning, and other household duties. They respectfully kept their distance from the active clinical arena. We all had our place, and that made our working environment a joy. The same *esprit de corps* we enjoyed many decades ago needs to return.

Reexamining the Status quo

While some resist new ideas and suggestions for change, others embrace them. Just like the fictional Marty McFly in the film *Back to the Future* (1985), ideas can move ahead of what is acceptable at the time. Marty discovered that his 1955 audience of teenagers could not appreciate 'Rock & Roll' before it became fashionable and widely accepted (although it was in 1955 that Chuck Berry signed a contract with Chess Records after he wrote "Maybelline"). Without some personal involvement, future trends are never easy to guess, although the politically expedient and the economical will always gain favour.

In the long term what you know, or how good you are as a nurse or doctor, may matter less to the progress of your career than you think. Your attitude, ideas, and relationship with others might shape it more. This is unlikely to change in the future.

If, like me, you are not respectful, obsequious, remorseful, or contrite enough in your attitude towards inspectors and regulators and their awesome power, you risk being sanctioned or removed. They do not see the removal of doctors and the good they do as an abuse of their statutory power. That is because they underestimate medical professionals as societal assets. As valuable assets doctors and nurses take decades to replace. Punitive GMC and PSA regulation therefore needs to be reviewed urgently.

Most doctors and nurses are self-sufficient, but inspectors and regulators will hesitate to acknowledge this, as it might undermine their position. When choosing test pilots and astronauts, one need only recruit those who possess the ability and knowledge for self-sufficiency. They need to be made of the 'right stuff'. The same principle applies to choosing students who will make competent doctors. They will then need teachers who can foster their independence with knowledge, expertise, experience, and wise clinical judgement. The stone on which they wrote this principle needs polishing.

Who gets to judge the dancing in the very popular BBC TV programme *Strictly Come Dancing*? Will they choose non-dancing lay people? Perhaps lawyers or accountants should do it? Is it possible that only professional dancers will make credible judges?

We allow MPTS tribunals to be composed of one lawyer, one lay person, and a GP. It is they who are chosen to judge the performance of long-established doctors and their skill, and to shape their future career prospects. Does this pass the same common sense test used to choose those qualified to judge dancing competitions? Composed of senior, experienced doctors, we can expect only a Medical Directorate to deliver justice to doctors using their clinical perspective.

For the future to be safe, we must regularly reexamine the status quo of medical bureaucracy. Is it 'fit for purpose' (to use one of their own well-worn corporate catchphrases)?

Trivial Pursuits

In 2019 there were only sixty GPs for every 100,000 of the UK population. This number reduced over the prior five-year period. Older GPs were retiring (for pension and tax reasons, and because of burnout and demoralisation), and younger ones dropped out of training schemes.

A survey of GP work undertaken by Pulse magazine (May 2019) revealed that GPs worked an eleven-hour day, with forty-one patient contacts on average. Half of the GPs surveyed felt that they were working in a way which compromised patient safety.

Some hospital doctors think the work of GPs is too trivial, boring, and laborious to inspire them intellectually. If we freed GPs from bureaucratic administration altogether, they might have more time for clinical medicine and surgery (although many genuinely enjoy the clinical content of general practice and its associated lifestyle). After having had their knowledge, clinical ability and judgement challenged, some could gain in self-esteem. If we delegate all the administrative roles of doctors, and allow minor medical conditions to be treated by nurses and paramedics, we might make the job of GPs more attractive.

Those trained to administer should do just that. We should leave medical secretaries, managers, and PAs to sift through paperwork, write letters, update computer screens, and action managerial decisions like referrals and appointments. NHS doctors could then spend more time with patients. Some might even elect to talk to their patients at greater length when necessary and come to know them better. This would emulate private practice culture. GPs might have more time to join a hospital team, teach students and nurses, and provide valuable clinical and social context. If they chose to, they could assist the surgeons who operate on their patients (as once many did before the NHS). This would turn the clock back to the all-private, pre-NHS days. The effect would be to make the job for some, instantly more interesting, intellectually more satisfying, and far less dispiriting. It would need a cultural change that could be strongly resisted.

Not all GPs choose medicine for its academic interest and clinical involvement. Lifestyle and social factors are just as important to many who now choose general practice as a career. For many years, the trend has been for junior doctors to choose general practice to get a better work life balance (pursuing hobbies, sports, running a business of their own, and more involvement with their family). Having no weekend or night work has enabled this.

Because they represent doctors' interests, the BMA are dutybound to resist replacing GPs with nurses and paramedics, as such changes would obviously reduce GP numbers. Those left (consultant GPs) would have to be capable of in-depth clinical involvement. The change would aid both job satisfaction for nurses and improve job satisfaction for those doctors tired of administration and quick-fix medicine.

Whatever happens, continuing in the way UK general practice now functions is not an option. Patients waiting two to three weeks for a face-to-face appointment, with patients allowed only ten to fifteen minutes for consultations to discuss only one topic, is second-rate. It is unacceptable and unfair to patients and GPs alike.

Future General Practice

The NHS lost over 700 GPs in the three years before 2022. These losses are causing serious medical service crises, but how are further losses to be stopped?

I would like to make some 'tongue-in-cheek' suggestions for the future of general practice in the UK, taken from how my own private general medical and cardiological practice functioned. Many of these suggestions already exist in the EU, where medical practice more closely resembles UK private practice. Most would be unthinkable unless they became politically expedient. In the UK some of my recommendations are beyond the medical bureaucratic event horizon, and are inconsistent with NHS culture. Here is my shortlist of twenty-five suggestions.

1. To create a consultant class of GP, supported by intelligent, motivated nurses and paramedics, trained especially for the job of minor clinical medicine (perhaps a three-year medical degree course).

2. All bureaucratic processes, like writing notes and documentation, to be passed to PAs, managers and secretaries.

3. Some GPs to adopt a hospital specialty with training in hospital medicine, surgery, 'obs. and gynae'.

4. Continuity of established doctor patient relationships to be regarded as a *sine qua non* of practise. Patients changing practices should ask how much continuity the new practice offers (see '7').

5. Improved availability. Some GP practices to open all day, 8:00am to 8:00pm, with selected ones open for twenty-four hours. This would make their services equivalent to some pharmacists. It would allow consulting times to expand beyond ten to fifteen minutes.

6. Every eligible patient to carry an official summary of their clinical notes (the NHS app is a start). This will allow every doctor other than their own, to brief themselves without delay. Patients can carry their clinical data on a mobile device. Any doctor undertaking an online or telephone consultation should review the details to improve safety.

7. Every patient should be able to change their GP without a registration problem, with access to doctors of their choice, NHS or 'private'. UK GP practices effectively 'possess' the patients on their list. This is out of step with all other professional practices. Patients should be free to move between doctors if they want. They should be free to choose doctors (private or NHS) with whom they can develop continuous, meaningful relationships, should they want.

8. The NHS should fund private GP consultations when NHS services are unavailable. A&E visits should not

be the first alternative.

9. Remuneration for doctors to include recognition of any specialised work they do.

10. CQC inspectors and regulators should be given a new role: to help maintain GP practice systems, not just issue judgements of inadequacy. Inspectors and regulators should facilitate housekeeping and maintenance improvements when found wanting. The CQC should adopt a supportive role, one that would improve practices rather than alienate them.

11. The CQC should not have any involvement in clinical issues. If allegations arise, a Medical Directorate should review them.

12. Nurses, paramedics and pharmacists to receive pay commensurate with their clinical work.

13. Every consulting GP to be allowed an accredited specialty, and remunerated at specialist rates. They could divide their day into routine, emergency, and specialist cases. Some hospital work would then become obligatory.

14. Doctor profiles (professional and personal) should be available to patients. Doctors with a personal interest or specialty should be available to patients who need their expertise, regardless of practice boundaries. An app would enable this.

15. Retiring doctors to upload their unproven ideas and unfinished projects to an open database, accessible to young doctors seeking research projects.

16. Doctors to have greater self-sufficiency, able to decide on the management of their practices, but be totally responsible for every clinical outcome.

17. Experienced, troubleshooting doctors to be sent to help

practices with waiting lists.

18. Practices voted down by patients, and agreed by a Medical Directorate, to be restaffed.

19. Charge some patients at the point of service if they repeatedly waste consulting time (for which there must be evidence). The lack of a token charge has contributed to the abuse of medical staff, especially by those who insist on exercising their rights.

20. Managers (and some doctors), inspectors, and regulators to be directly responsible for patients who die or are harmed, because of a long waiting list. Any adverse result of a statutory intervention contrary to Medical Directorate advice should be the subject of an investigation.

21. A Medical Directorate tribunal should arbitrate between practitioners, managers, and regulators when clinical matters are in dispute.

22. Medical practitioners must keep control of their practice and retain primary clinical responsibility unless proven harm has come to a patient. No doctor's practice should be closed or threatened with closure, without first being reviewed by patients and the Medical Directorate.

23. Learning, rather than retribution, should be the guiding principle behind all inspections and regulation. The public cannot afford to lose doctors or their practices when education alone would repair their functioning. The removal of one doctor from a practice will have a greater detrimental effect on the public than removing many inspectors.

24. Annual appraisals and regular revalidations that promote education and standards are essential. Their current format is superfluous, functioning as they do

as corporate data collection exercises, and a means for the GMC to gain income through certification. They are not medically expedient and should change.

25. The sovereign duty of doctors and nurses is essential to Western society. The rules that govern medical regulators, including the CQC and their inspectors, must change to reflect this. We should re-task them to offer suggestions and advice, not punishment or restrictive orders. They must be liable for personal and corporate disciplinary action should any of their orders or actions prove detrimental to any medical professional or any patient.

Some Other Political Considerations

Accountancy drives most corporate decision making. The NHS is no exception. Politicians must listen to the voice of financial controllers. Without them, corporations risk failure. For sound financial reasons, they will argue for more GP physician associates, nurse practitioners, more AI, and fewer doctors (GPs) in the future.

In order to rekindle our image as dedicated medical professionals, it would help to bring back willing retired doctors for a few sessions every week. They could help reduce patient backlogs, introduce continuity, and bring the benefits of long experience. Important aspects of corporate inertia, standardisation, certification and red tape would have to change in order to facilitate its implementation.

Will doctors in the UK ever resign *en masse* in order to take back control of their medical practice? As the medical regulatory corporations know full well, doctors and nurses are too insecure and too dedicated to their work to contemplate this, unless pushed to extremes. Not so our dental colleagues. Their 2006 contract was punitive. Based on a points system, it resulted in a lot of extra work for no added income. Many dentists now refuse NHS patients, and when they take them on, they find many with advanced disease from a lack of dental care. They can then offer only extractions and dentures. This is not what one might expect in a first-world country! No government has changed their contract or increased funding since 2006. We are now witnessing the widespread resignation of dentists from the NHS.

It is easy to disregard the discontented voices of nurses, doctors, and dentists. Politicians might take these voices to be the disingenuous carping of advantaged people, few of whom identify with the average man. The result of ignoring the views of medical staff, underpaying them, and giving them no respect for their skills, judgement and lifesaving decision-making, can only be to disgruntle, demean, and demoralise them. That has already happened and is unlikely to change in the future without better staffing, funding, and regulatory changes that give NHS decision-making power back to medical professionals.

Patients need to influence plans for medical practice. Patients are voters, and outnumber doctors by 2000: 1 (perhaps why politicians can sideline doctors). Our health system should first satisfy the basic medical demands of patients. Instead of satisfying their demands, the government may find it more expedient to lower their expectations.

In the current era, medical bureaucratic supremacy is distinct from that which I first encountered when practising medicine. Clinical medicine seemed to work well because patient welfare was in the hands of only those dedicated to it, and those who knew most about it. Whipps Cross Hospital in 1966 needed only one Director of Nursing ('Matron'), one senior consultant doctor, and one general manager (with limited staff) to run the 800-bedded hospital. Managers had a simple brief. That was to fulfil the requirements of doctors and nurses caring for patients. The system was good enough to generate *esprit de corps*. Patients would now benefit if we selected the best from the past, and applied it to the future.

We got a glimpse of the same old spirit and respect for doctors and nurses during the COVID-19 pandemic. Ministers of the state actually declared that they were deferring decisions to medical science. It fell to medical scientists to interpret clinical information in politically expedient ways. They made some serious mistakes. One was not to stop air travel from China early enough. Another was not to heed the lessons of the 1918 influenza pandemic, and what had recently happened in Europe.

No discussion of the lessons learned from the influenza epidemic of 1918 to 1919 took place in public. Fifty to one hundred million people died worldwide on that occasion. The information might have induced panic.

Dr. James Niven, who was Medical Officer for Health in Manchester on that occasion, published his observations (Report on the Epidemic of Influenza in Manchester, 1918 to 1919). He advised:

- The closure of schools (although the dispersal of the virus in homes was more significant).
- Social distancing by avoiding crowds.
- The isolation of the sick.
- The cleansing of utensils and towels used by the sick.
- The wearing of masks on public transport (if the public

agreed).
* Regular hand washing.

Going Solo

One acceptable way to avoid corporate control is for doctors to copy UK dentists and start their own practices. It might increase in the future, if the CQC would allow it. In keeping with the corporate NHS, they prefer group practices and their management structure. They believe in safety in numbers. Any doctor starting his own practice will be responsible for his own fate, his own self-esteem, and the welfare of his patients. He will need demonstrable competence, affability, and a natural understanding of his patients. For the majority, solo private practice would require too much financial commitment, and be far too adventurous. Dentists do it, so why not doctors?

How many doctors would now be as confident as were their pre-NHS forefathers to start their own practice? They were personally responsible for their professional future. I have only met two doctors in the last fifty years who qualified for the role. The alternative is for doctors to resign themselves to being corporate employees, comfortable with group support, and happy to observe every guideline, regulation and directive imposed on them by an employing authority.

Are independent solo practices such a good thing? Some patients value the continuity they bring and the type of relationship they can have with one doctor. After Shipman, the absence of peer review has meant that solo practises are now regarded as dangerous.

A Duty to Teach Medicine?

Experienced older doctors and nurses should teach. I believe those with forty to fifty years of practise experience should pass on a few tips to younger professionals. Such information may be out-of-date, but can be too valuable to be forgotten (my book, *The Doctor's Apprentice. The Art and Science of Medicine*, is my contribution). Unfortunately there is no system for older doctors to give masterclasses. Once you are out of the teaching hospital loop, you are out for good.

I found being a lecturer frustrating. Students rightly ask medical lecturers, 'How do you know that?' and, 'What is your evidence for that?' These questions are likely to annoy those with decades of experience. In order to fend off annoyance, some teachers become aloof, arrogant, angry, didactic or simply unpleasant. There is no justification for inappropriate behaviour, whether it be from a five-year-old child, or a seventy-five-year-old physician. Many will find the challenge of teaching enjoyable and worthwhile. Some will enjoy the kudos and the attention of young followers.

In the late eighteenth century, at St. George's, Hyde Park Corner, London, the anatomist and surgeon John Hunter had suffered angina pectoris. He announced, 'My life is in the hands of any rascal that choose to annoy or tease me!' He collapsed and died in 1793 at a meeting of St George's Board of Governors at which he was involved in a heated discussion over the admission of students.

David Dighton

Doctors as Patient Advocates

Retired doctors could play many important roles. They could help dissatisfied patients, especially those who need more time for explanation than UK medical practice now allows. I still get asked to act as a medical tutor and advocate to friends being assessed and managed by their doctors. If dissatisfied or unsure, they telephone me for my comments and unofficial appraisal. They sometimes find it valuable to discuss their problems with an experienced friend. At least I can tell them what questions to ask their doctor. The role allows patients to gain a better perspective of their condition and their likely journey through the medical maze. Many have known me to support wise management and to question inappropriate management.

I once considered helping staff on hospital wards during Christmas and New Year. As an old doctor, I could never have provided the documentation deemed necessary by bureaucrats. I never had scissors sharp enough to cut through their red tape!

Regulators, Inspectors, and 'Two Cultures' (C.P. Snow)

The GMC and CQC are replete with those who have studied humanities. Few of them have studied science. The medical profession and regulators thus represent two cultures. The bureaucratic view of medical practice has it that corporate legal considerations are as important, if not more important, than scientific ones. Without a scientific education, what else should we expect from them? Some who work for them will hold tacit, insupportable presumptions about medical practice which will need extirpating in the future. Here are a few:

- That clinical experience means nothing.
- That certification confirms competence.
- That the standardisation of medical practice is a basic requirement.
- That general rules apply to every individual.
- That all doctors contribute equally to patients.
- That guidelines can be used as immutable rules and used to test compliance.
- That patients' opinions have no more validity than hearsay.
- The only information required to judge a doctor's performance is documentary evidence, and third-party opinion, not metainformation.
- That bureaucrats have the right to override patient confidentiality (by getting High Court orders), and can examine any patient's confidential notes without their permission.
- That patients should trust bureaucrats more than doctors and nurses.
- That bureaucrats are fit for the guardianship of medical practice, and that doctors and nurses are questionably qualified for the role.
- That their spying on doctors and nurses is acceptable, if they deem it necessary in the public interest.

What might shock patients most, I suspect, is that some medical bureaucrats regard doctors and nurses as potentially dangerous criminals, until proven otherwise. Patients who trust doctors with their lives might find this incredulous, unless they too have had experience of regulators.

Receptionists as Valuable Gatekeepers

Whether a medical receptionist, a bouncer at a nightclub, or a customs official at an international border, the ability to judge people and discriminate between them is crucial to their performance. Medical receptionists and those who man emergency telephone services are critical gatekeepers. This is far from a trivial role. We ask them to judge clinical urgency. That is a lot to ask of someone who has not been medically trained. Many have a natural gift for it, and seem to understand people better than most. We could further train those with this talent to improve their patient management skills. Because of the knowledge they possess, nurses or paramedics often make ideal receptionists, although some will think it beneath them. An effective receptionist will structure a doctor's working day in order of clinical priority, but a poor one will cause some patients to suffer unacceptably. It is time to take the role of medical receptionist more seriously.

The Future of Nurses in Medical Practice

Nurses in training need support. Many will need a bursary to allow them to live a modest life while studying. They may need nurseries for their children and free meals while on duty, and should not have to pay for parking.

Many retired nurses would be happy to return to duty in times of patient overload. At the moment there are so many bureaucratic restrictions that they could easily become de-incentivised.

Nurses and paramedics are usually modest about their skills, some of which include clinical assessment and preliminary diagnosis. They work well with checklists, but can outgrow them as they learn to use metainformation wisely from experience. Many are effective in managing chronic disease cases; some have a facility for working in acute and emergency situations. At present their range of knowledge and skills limits them in the UK. The remedy is to offer them medical courses that match their learning abilities. Some capable nurses and paramedics could progress to full medical qualification, while others will be happy to train for nurse practitioner status in specific fields.

There is a trial about to take place: nurses using virtual reality goggles. This is being introduced by the NHS department of transformation. Their consultations will be recorded, saving time on notetaking (they spend half of their time on paperwork), with data streamed to appropriate doctors when needed. How patients will take to seeing nurses wearing

VR goggles awaits to be seen. If patients were to conclude that UK medicine is being depersonalised further by computer enthusiasts, they could be correct.

Many paramedics have already proven their lifesaving capability in acute trauma and A&E scenarios. They can stabilise deteriorating patients using intubation, ventilation, intravenous fluids and resuscitation. They may lack the ability to interpret unusual or confusing presentations, but with help, they could make reliable diagnoses and develop clinical judgement. Many will be eligible for medical apprenticeship.

Who Else Might Run the NHS?

Would the NHS be any different if medical insurers or private health provider corporations, ran it? Or would this simply be swapping one corporation for another?

For any corporation to claim success, its shareholders, and most of its customers or patients, need to be satisfied. They all have a problem. The standardisation all large organisations require can anonymously service the average case, but will not easily satisfy individuals with unusual problems. This conflicts with the work of practising doctors and nurses, whose focus is always on the problems of individuals.

Apart from delivering medical services, the NHS has nothing to do with profit, and a lot to do with gaining political advantage. The public needs to feel grateful to encourage voting. With politicians and their managers steadily losing their grip on NHS finances, the NHS risks being handed over to profit-motivated medical insurers and other private medical providers. A key issue for doctors and nurses is whether they would be better off financially with corporate insurance managers and their accountants, or bureaucrats working for the government? The constraints imposed on doctors by every corporate business would start innocently, but get tighter if profits fell. If the NHS executives choose to delegate clinical work to private corporations, they could control them by introducing renewable licences. They could threaten rescinding them should they not get what they want.

The top priority for all business corporations is profit, including those who might come to run the NHS. Without profit a business corporation running the NHS would see their shareholders dumping shares. A medical corporation running the NHS or private hospitals would have a healthy income; their problem would be to control the expenses. They might aggressively sanction staff performing overly expensive procedures. They might reduce what is unprofitable (research, and the treatment of rare and chronic diseases), and maximise the profitable procedures like hip and knee replacements, CABGs, and angioplasty.

As a sneaky political gambit, in the best tradition of *Yes, Minister* (the TV series), the government might just let other corporations have a go at running the NHS. If they failed it would teach doctors and the public to respect government bureaucracy. They could then proclaim the need to return us all to a refashioned NHS, with even more constraints, ones which the public would have to accept with grace. If the profit-based companies succeeded, the government could take credit for their wise delegation.

David Dighton

Future Efficiency, Productivity, and Patients

Knowing they could not cope with the demand of allcomers, NHS controllers long ago decided to use private hospitals to treat some elective and chronic cases. They offered NHS contracts to Virgin Health and other companies. If this is part of a long-term, NHS sell-off plan, it would leave the NHS with only emergency and acute medical care. These services would remain a well-deserved source of pride for the NHS.

Targets for shortening waiting lists and improving doctor availability, now focus the minds of NHS bureaucrats. We had short waiting lists and unquestioned doctor availability in the 1960s, well before the appearance of any overbearing bureaucracy and exponential population growth. The increased demand from a larger population (52.37 million in 1960; 67.44 million in 2022), only partly explains the diminishing availability of medical services. Since the 1960s, medical bureaucracy has organised medical services into lumped-together practices (polyclinics and hub-hospitals justified by financial efficiency), disjointed GP and social services, and a system that is dysfunctional for patients because of reduced availability. Hospital services do not link up with social services, and almost no doctor patient continuity now exists. What medical services we now have do not deserve the same kudos that the NHS had in the 1960s. NHS bureaucracy has failed. The only options are a complete change of regime (and culture), or death of the system and the handover to private enterprise.

The fractionation of the medical profession in the UK by specialisation has made it more difficult for patients to find an appropriate doctor. Specialisation has restricted overall functioning, even for NHS GPs, whose scope of work has contracted over recent decades. After qualifying in 1966, I received training in hospital medicine, some surgery, A&E (then casualty), anaesthetics, obstetrics, and cardiology. On a desert island, I could still perform these functions. I wonder if modern graduates would feel confident enough to work there, or feel trained enough to survive outside of their certificated roles. Hopefully they will never have to.

Having experienced them firsthand, my guess is that many old doctors and patients would support the return of (NHS) cottage hospitals. In effect they have returned, but as small private independent hospitals. They once suited the diverse skills of family doctors and were liked by patients, who found them friendly, efficient, and convenient.

A network of NHS polyclinics with a few beds could provide the same facilities as cottage hospitals. If GPs could admit and care for their own patients with specialist support, general practice would become so much more interesting and rewarding for some. Many patients would find the resulting continuity invaluable.

Hospital Practice Recommendations

Foremost, hospital beds need to be freed for acute medical use. Because nobody recovers quickly from any debilitating medical condition or surgery, the NHS thought convalescent homes necessary. Reintroducing them again as once suggested by Alan Milburn the health secretary in 2000 (BMJ. 2000; 320(7232): 401), would serve the valuable purpose of freeing acute hospital beds and helping to reduce waiting lists. If they thought of refurbishing offices, hotels and large buildings for the purpose, that would represent urgent wartime thinking.

A formidable hierarchy of corporate managers, regulators, and politicians now runs NHS hospital practice. They harbour a morbid delusion: that they know all they need to know about medical practice. The delusion partly explains why the NHS has become increasingly dysfunctional.

What defines medical dysfunctionality? A lack of joined-up care from hospitals, GPs and social services; log-jams of patients waiting for investigations, operations and treatment for cancer; patients not being seen quickly enough, or investigated and diagnosed early enough for their clinical priority. These are all signs of medical service dysfunction. For the richer few, the UK private sector does a much better job.

Because illness knows no 'right time', patients will present in clusters, and almost never in an even stream. This means the NHS can only achieve functionality for short periods, and then only by luck if understaffed.

The views and needs of experienced doctors and nurses providing the service and the views of patients and their relatives need to be given priority. Otherwise we can expect

211

many more Mid. Staffs., and Shrewsbury and Telford maternity scandals. Hospitals must respond to local needs and are best managed locally.

Hospital efficiency depends on staff capability. *Esprit de corps* is essential and improves with technical capability and successful patient handling. Every clinical team needs to be directed by an experienced, knowledgeable, and respected senior doctor. Teams of capable staff can inspire healthy competition between departments and between hospitals. Healthy competition was once a feature at London teaching hospitals. As a London hospital graduate, I still find it difficult to comprehend that 'The London' was amalgamated with our once arch-rival, Bart's! We challenged them, rowing on the Thames, and on rugby pitches. At St. George's, we specialised in slow heart rhythms and left the tachycardias to Bart's cardiologists. These distinctions were once a source of collective enthusiasm and pride.

Imposed office duties, whether in hospital or general practice, serve to demean our medical status. Doctors should never waste their valuable time on office tasks that feed the corporation with management data. This is a job for secretaries and PAs. No director of a business corporation would ever get involved in such activities, nor should any doctor or nurse. On the same basis, medical staff should never deal directly with NHS bureaucrats. The focus of doctors and nurses should never drift from matters that concern patient morbidity and mortality.

Hospitals need the equivalent of medical commanding officers to preside over managers. Only senior, experienced doctors and nurses, with time and inclination for housekeeping matters, should contemplate getting involved. Those managerial functionaries who run hospitals should take their lead from those with clinical expertise, not *vice versa*. As long as politicians object to such rearrangements (and they will, to protect their political position), the NHS will continue its downhill path (even less time for patients, much longer waiting lists, and many more management executives employed to solve the problems). Since politicians are rarely in office for long, they will be happy to pass on this poisoned chalice.

Considerable but inactive human resources exist. Retired nurses who no longer hold certification, and retired doctors, should sometimes be co-opted in times of need (like Territorial Army soldiers). At least one bureaucrat thought of this during the COVID-19 pandemic.

Medical care has become a basic right for all citizens in most democratic societies. Without a healthy nation, societies will break down. Defence and public safety are important government priorities, but for most individuals, health takes equal priority.

The dedication of NHS medical staff has always deserved applause. The case I make here against the need for so many medical bureaucrats found support during the COVID-19 pandemic. Hospital staff worked well without corporate managers. For a time they were absent, and could not command medical staff to dance to their scripted managerial directives. Hospital bureaucrats went home and put their feet up, while independent, self-motivated doctors and nurses showed their mettle. This was not a time for timewasting management gobbledygook, but then there never has been!

The Need for a Medical Directorate

I am not the first to suggest it, but I strongly support the proposal for a medical directorate, set up by the Royal colleges to supersede all the functions of the GMC, CQC, and PSA whenever the clinical actions of doctors need review and need to be judged. It would fail in its purpose unless beyond government bureaucratic control. It would require its own statutory authority independent of the PSA, leaving doctors, not lawyers, to review and judge all medical matters.

Any medical professional who has engaged with the PSA, GMC, or CQC will understand the need. The staff of these corporations cannot claim any in-depth understanding of the work of doctors, nurses, or clinical practice. They lack the appropriate educational background and clinical experience. Their ethos is not appropriate; it is legal, not medical. They correctly state that their job is to apply the law. They should then only become involved when the proposed medical directorate has detected criminal behaviour. From a clinical standpoint, their functioning can represent the insolence of power: power without responsibility, and power applied without sufficient knowledge and clinical experience. Without insolence, how can they think to involve themselves in the assessment of doctors and nurses, and apply the law safely, fairly, and proportionately?

Hospitals need to give priority to clinicians who know what medical services they need. They have appointed doctors to NHS medical directorates run predominantly by bureaucrats, but these are separate from what I propose to be the functioning of an independent medical directorate. Those doctors who now staff NHS medical directorates will have bureaucratic aspirations and, like other bureaucrats, may view the culture, opinions, and judgements of practising clinicians as marginal.

Since the nationalisation of medicine in the UK in 1948, political expediency has assumed priority over medical issues. The leadership that Peter Lees suggests (CEO and medical director, Faculty of Medical Leadership and Management) is one that must come from those with sufficient medical knowledge. Would he and the RCP be brave enough to support the removal of corporate government leadership, and replace it with medical leadership (as occurred temporarily during the COVID-19 pandemic)?

A Vital Experiment: Hospitals run by Doctors and Nurses

Consider the thesis: 'hospital bureaucracy is mostly superfluous, obstructive, and dangerous to the welfare of patients'. I suggest a trial to prove it: hospitals administered solely by nurses and doctors, with bureaucrats engaged only in housekeeping duties, and no authority to interfere in any matter that involves patient handling, care, or management.

Politicians are smart. They all know that health provision is a poisoned chalice. Why don't they make the medical profession completely responsible for the delivery of healthcare? They would have a win, win, win situation. Politicians, medical professionals and patients would all benefit.

Should the GMC and MPTS be replaced?

Medical Practitioner Tribunals (undertaken by the MPTS) are supposedly independent of the GMC, except their rules, regulations, and guidelines are all dictated by the GMC. Without a dedicated medical directorate with statutory authority, crucial clinical issues, clinical common sense, and the wisdom of clinical experience will continue to get overlooked. The MPTS does its best to be fair to doctors, but is it fair to their tribunal members?

They have several specially trained legal chairs to choose from, and a lawyer always leads their tribunals. They also have 300 lay and medical associates to choose from to fill the other seats. Many of their laypeople have legal degrees or have experience in bureaucratic roles. Most doctors they use are NHS GPs, steeped in NHS culture, with many others trained in psychology, psychiatry, and gynaecology. There are very few practising hospital physicians and surgeons available to them. In fact, very few doctors they call on will be in full-time practice, with an understanding of the work conditions and constraints that all practising doctors face. There is an equivalent to employing lawyers, laypeople, and GPs to judge doctors who face allegations at medical tribunals (MPTS): call a plumber when your electricity supply fails!

Courts of law function on an adversarial interchange between two opposing representatives. The binary verdict of guilty or not guilty can be based only on the documentary evidence presented. The assumption of innocence and the principle of 'reasonable doubt' should always be involved since clinicians make judgements differently (see my book, *The Doctor's Apprentice*). Each clinician will discuss the weight of evidence and its likelihood of being correct rather than assuming its validity (often assumed) when alternative diagnoses and management plans are discussed. These differences expose a systemic fault in legalistic MPTS tribunal functioning. The adversarial legal process does not reflect the clinical decision-making process, especially when hearsay evidence or metainformation is regarded as unacceptable. Both feature strongly in clinical decision-making. For justice to be done, it must involve experienced practitioners judging the reasoning and weight of factors used in the clinical decision-making. They did not try to do this during any of my appearances before MPTS tribunals.

Claiming to protect the public from medical risk (especially from the actions of doctors), using the judgements of a lawyer, laypersons, and GPs is not possible. GPs do not handle clinical risk. They identify then refer patients at risk to those doctors experienced at managing it. Lawyers and laypeople know nothing about active risk assessment in clinical settings. Who else but doctors involved with daily clinical risk assessment could assess the risks other doctors take? If tribunals (as composed above) assume they can, injustices must result. I wonder how many doctors they have unfairly removed from practice as a result. My guess is that those featured by media outlets are but the tip of an iceberg.

The GMC is unfit to try doctors who have not harmed patients, and who have no substantiated complaints against them. Only when allegations of criminal acts have been received will their adversarial legal setup be appropriate.

The MPTS trial system allows accused doctors to request

their own experts to report on the allegations. The independent medical experts are not required to know the scene of the alleged action or the circumstances at first hand. They may thus avoid making a personal assessment of doctors on trial, their practice, patients, and individual circumstances. We may then see them as impartial and independent. Unfortunately, avoiding metainformation is a potential source of error when a true understanding of a doctor's work is essential. The past clinical experience and performance of a doctor, his academic prowess and seniority, and the comments of his patients, if taken as hearsay (synonymous with 'totally unreliable', or evidence of no useful value), will deny tribunals the perspective they need for wise decision-making. These are the restrictions unfairly applied when an adversarial legal process tries to judge clinical allegations without medical knowledge. To assess noncriminal doctors and their actions in this way lacks common sense and fairness.

Without a visiting team to review the content of a doctor's work, how can a fair appraisal of a doctor's work be made? The views of his staff, colleagues, and patients are all of crucial importance. No human evaluation can be complete without an inspection of the *locus in quo*. Without this the MPTS cannot consider the existence of exceptional patients or exceptional circumstances. Because they are not clinicians, we cannot expect them to appreciate the wide natural variance of patients, the different ways they present to us, and how they all need to be managed differently. This variance makes the practice of medicine complex, and one step beyond the merely complicated (see *Hayek's theory on complexity and knowledge.* Stefano Fiori: https://doi.org/10.1080/13501780903128548). Patient understanding and handling, doctor patient exposure, and continuity all need to be considered. The MPTS tribunal considered none of these in my case. How often are they considered in other cases?

If losing one doctor from providing a medical service has more relevance to the public than the loss of one lawyer or regulator, the MPTS and GMC must learn to gain a wider perspective, some clinical understanding, and to be more considerate.

Leaving the judgement of doctors to an NHS GP, a layperson and a lawyer cannot hope to reflect public need. Let's put it to a vote. Ask a random public group: *'You have the choice of losing a lawyer, a layperson with bureaucratic experience, or a practising doctor from service. Which one would you choose?'* The answers will suggest whether the GMC/MPTS is fit for purpose.

The purpose of MPTS tribunals is to judge a doctor's compliance with GMC rules. Their corporate authority to guard the safety of patients and the reputation of the medical profession needs scrutiny. A 360-degree human evaluation (required of doctors in their appraisals), with a focus on remediation not persecution and prosecution, is now essential. While they keep the legal right to pursue enforcement, urgent change is necessary. They must realise the political value of the human asset lost whenever one doctor is denied clinical work.

One cannot standardise the art of medicine or how to deal with clinical risk. Therefore, one cannot reliably judge it using any of the fixed laws, rules, and regulations required for standardisation. Even those who have not practiced medicine or nursing can (delete 'surely) appreciate this. Is it intelligent for the GMC and MPTS and their lawyers to judge a doctor who has coped with an individual medical problem, knowing that the features may not conform to the usual? Corporate legal involvement should be withheld if no harm has come to a patient, especially if the doctor (as in my case) has the full support of his patient. The focus should be on peer review, advice, and further education, not persecution. It is understandable that our regulators, given the rules we charge them to protect, will want to act in a failsafe manner. They must thus impose sanctions that avoid their culpability.

The ill-informed, the stupid, and those who lack the required breadth of knowledge will rely on what is usual, not the exceptional. Usual standards and prescribed methods, dictated from corporate head-offices may make a baked bean factory efficient, but these methods are of little use in the consulting room, operating theatre, or catheter laboratory. These are places where clinical competence involves handling variation and change, risk assessment, and constant reevaluation. These are places where regular changes in direction may be needed to favour patient safety and survival. What regulators will find difficult to acknowledge is that these dynamic factors often exist, and differ considerably between patients. For those without experience of this, wise decision-making by those whose job it is to sit in judgment on doctors will be impossible.

The CQC

The CQC does a commendable job protecting the public from ineffective and dangerous medical and nursing practices. Their judgement rests on important housekeeping factors like the safety of medical and fire equipment, hygiene, and fire escape procedures. What they are not qualified to do is judge the ability, knowledge and functional adequacy of doctors engaging with patients. Their inspection teams will sometimes include a corporate-savvy NHS GP, but can he safely judge doctors who work in other medical fields, those who work privately, or those who do not share his NHS culture, ideas or attitudes? I ran a private cardiac screening unit for decades, so what standard of appraisal could I have expected from an NHS GP or CQC inspector? The adequacy of their inspection teams to judge more specialised medical practices needs review.

During their inspections CQC inspectors spend a lot of time reading the standardised corporate-based protocols produced by each practice. Many practice managers copy these from reliable internet sources. Few doctors and nurses have any inclination to compose them for themselves.

They train CQC inspectors to be corporate-minded and checklist oriented. This ensures they gather data in a standardised manner. Their checkboxes cover important areas of practise: person-centred care, dignity and respect, consent, safety, safeguarding from abuse, food and drink, premises and equipment, complaints, governance, staffing, and duty of candour. Any discussion of topics beyond these will make them zone out. If they take on more corporate staff at head office, they will doubtless invent more checkboxes. This will prolong inspection visits, and keep doctors away from their valuable work longer.

A CQC inspector once suggested I put security bars on the windows of my first-floor consulting room, just in case a psychiatric patient jumped out. I declined, but said that I would never again allow a psychiatrist to work on the first floor!

The CQC once condemned my practice. They thought it seriously unsafe. They issued me with an urgent warning notice. This gave me forty-eight hours to come up with answers to pages of questions they thought were of urgent concern. Because I had no 'hand-washing signs' over my wash basins, they judged my infection control to be poor. The implication was that my patients faced a grave infection risk when they visited me. They must have assumed that my staff and patients did not know how and when to wash their hands! They ignored the fact that I did not undertake surgery. The basis of their argument was 'you never can tell', and 'you never know what might happen tomorrow' (I only saw one infected post-injection site in forty years). Had any of my students used equivalent logic, or showed an equivalent talent for risk assessment, I would have dismissed them as unsuitable to practise medicine. Yet the CQC can come with the statutory power to command doctors, some with no discernible ability to judge the knowledge and ability of the professionals they regulate. Why should they care? Their job is to collect data as evidence, and complete checklists.

When donkeys command lions, and fools command the wise, they will usually miss any irony. The elephant usually present at CQC inspections would like to ask a question. Why should highly trained, experienced medical professionals need to respect them? Most CQC inspectors are reasonable and helpful, and are worthy of having patient safety as their priority. A few are arrogant and disrespectful and create antipathy.

Like the GMC, the CQC can regard GMC and NICE guidelines as immutable. That is neither the spirit nor the intention of NICE guidelines. The CQC and GMC will not discuss the point, since it is academic and rhetorical. The validity of their training and their clinical assumptions are also not open for discussion. I know they have the law on their side, but does that condone invalid assumptions? When bureaucrats deal with other bureaucrats, they will make complete sense to one another (cultural resonance); when medical professionals deal with bureaucrats, they must expect dissonance and no medical sense.

As a cardiologist (who very long ago spent two to three years as a principal GP), I was held in contempt by the CQC for undertaking 'general practice' (delete comma). They must have thought, that as an MRCP, I was qualified only for general hospital medicine, not general practice. For them, it was simply a matter of certification. I would question whether the content of GP work and the patients they see has changed since I last did such work, although I was last a GP in 1970, before being appointed as a British Heart Foundation research fellow in cardiology at St. George's Hospital (London, Hyde Park Corner).

On one occasion a CQC medical inspector referred me to the GMC for what he took to be my GP-related clinical management decisions. A few of my decisions affronted him from his perspective as a lecturer in general practice. Some were clearly beyond his expertise, but all were the subject of directives issued to GPs. His rule-based, guideline-restricted mind could not countenance the possibility of low-dose warfarin dosage being effective or prudent in an elderly, easily-bruised patient. We also disagreed about GP guidelines for the routine use of antibiotics in upper respiratory tract infections (coughs and sore throats). Although worried about sepsis, his view was that we should mostly withhold them. Having managed many cases of septicaemia in ITU, I did not agree without reservation. He took my discordance as a sign of ignorance and irreverence. In academic medicine, one must constantly challenge dogma, and test hard and fast rules with new and contrary evidence. His function as a lecturer was to teach rules, not to question them. He proved himself to be a lecturer, but not an academic.

Given his blinkered mind, I am sure the CQC regarded him as good at his job. Our views diverged so much that I proposed we agreed to differ. He took my adversarial academic medical approach as evidence of my unwillingness to comply. The PSA were later to use the same prosaic argument against me (see Appendix 2). When in conflict with regulatory processes, progress requires freethinking people to examine their dogma.

This inspector also examined many of my patient notes without permission from me or my patients. That was a step too far for this pompous pedant. While sitting on his high horse, he failed to convince me that general practice required the same intellectual approach needed by hospital doctors. I had no wish to emulate his churlishness by reporting him to the GMC. There has never been a place for either pious or petty people in my life or in medical practice!

CQC inspectors failed to consider important metadata about my practice (no check boxes for such information). My cardiac practice must have prevented many cardiac infarctions and strokes through the early detection of atheroma (artery 'furring'), but they were never interested. How could they justify ignoring these vital life and death issues? They obviously thought this was less important than the absence of 'Wash Your Hands' signs over my washbasins? Their lack of clinical perspective caused them to miss the whole purpose of my medical practice. Should the CQC continue to employ laypersons, nurses, lawyers and GPs to inspect hospitals and specialist practices like mine? On second thoughts, who else would want the job?

There will always be an intellectual gulf between those trained in science and those who studied the humanities (see C. P. Snow's *Two Cultures*). Because most bureaucrats have no scientific or medical education beyond the most elementary, they risk compromising any healthcare system they run. Few Ministers for Health have held a medical degree, and those who sit in the driving seats of the GMC and CQC corporate machines are mostly lawyers, capable of driving in a legal direction but not in a medical direction. They will struggle to get an accurate picture of a doctor's work, and it is foolhardy for them to attempt it without technical knowledge and clinical experience. As Mariana Mazzucato has pointed out (*The Big Con*, 2023, Allen Lane), government departments and corporations risk infantilisation when they refer all their technical decisions to outside consulting agencies.

Measures of the danger medical bureaucrats present to the medical profession are their unwillingness to acknowledge either their lack of clinical perspective and understanding, or the importance of clinical metainformation. All their false assumptions go unchallenged and their false conclusions about medical practice will continue until we staff them differently. Not much has changed in political power dynamics over the last century. Some donkeys still command lions.

An analogy with sport will illustrate how plain facts, like those relied on by both the CQC and GMC, are not enough to paint a complete picture. Every tennis and football match will end with a score, but does the score reflect how the game was played? The score alone cannot reflect how the game was fought, what struggles took place, and the worthiness of each player. Was it won by the positive actions of the winners or the failures of the losers? Every detail is essential if a professional evaluation of the game is to be made. Metainformation is clearly crucial to the in-depth understanding of dynamic situations. Taking it into account is the only basis for making fair and balanced conclusions.

I contend that neither the CQC, the GMC, nor the expert witnesses they rely on are interested in gathering and interpreting appropriate clinical metadata. If their proceedings were under the control of a Medical Directorate, valuable clinical metadata would be deemed essential for clinical interpretation. Fairer judgements would then be more likely to result for doctors and nurses.

In the future the law should change to give the CQC and GMC no involvement where clinical matters are the issue, especially when any consideration of clinical risk is involved. Their concerns should be legal ones only, and appropriate only when a patient has been harmed or has died. Who other than the members of a medical directorate could be trusted to judge a doctor's effect on a patient's morbidity and mortality? These are the only matters of importance to patients, and the only necessary preoccupations for those who practise medicine.

There is insufficient evidence to support the view that medical bureaucracy alone has improved patient safety, created effective medical practice, or improved public regard for the medical profession. Bureaucrats will disagree, so let's see their evidence. We will rely only on the most rigorous science-based methods to assess the value of their roles. Knowing they are unlikely to survive this challenge unscathed, their vehement resistance can be expected.

Epilogue

Those privileged to practise medicine and nursing hold a special place in society, where the state of health and quality of life of our fellow humans can be attended to, improved, and protected. Like food, air and water, most humans regard medical practice as indispensable. Medical practice has always been more than just a service co-opted by politicians to buy votes and to provide jobs for their bureaucrats. In the hearts of most, it is a sacrosanct discipline with sovereign status. Those who disagree should take a moment to consider life without medical professionals and carers.

Having retired before any bureaucrat could do their worst (something that soon followed), I am now resigned to watch history unfold, with bureaucrats and regulators exerting more of their untutored influence on patients, doctors and nurses. It is nothing new to know that the nature of bureaucracy is to imprison us in an iron cage (*Stahlhartes Gehäuse*, Max Weber, 1864 to 1920). This is something medical bureaucrats have successfully achieved in the UK. It is bureaucracy that has put the medical profession and UK clinical services into crisis.

UK medical bureaucrats now control many aspects of

medical practice, but worse is to come. They are now poised to interfere in the doctor patient relationship. Rule-based as they must be to function without medical knowledge or experience, they are plotting a path across quicksand. As they come to know the controlling and dispassionate purpose of medical bureaucracy that does little to improve their health, lifestyle, and longevity, patients will hopefully help doctors and nurses reduce bureaucratic interference. Can doctors and nurses afford to wait for this to happen? Even if bureaucrats lose some power, political elites will insist on their rebirth. While someone needs to manage the national health corporation, doctors and all medical professionals have a major duty to protect historic, mutually beneficial doctor patient relationships from bureaucratic interference.

It is ridiculous to think that anyone other than those who have mastered its science and art could presume to interfere with medicine as a scientific, experience-based discipline. Yet our regulators, with statutory powers and a flair for inductive logic and guesswork, insolently insist they can. Since its nationalisation in 1948, those trained in law, politics and business management have directed and controlled the NHS and how doctors and nurses can perform. That should not be allowed to continue unchanged.

Bureaucrats and regulators made my final two years of practice frustrating and pointless. I chose to rebuke them while fully aware of the inevitable consequences. I achieved my fifty-three year clinical record with no complaints from over 20,000 patients, so I would have much to be proud of, had pride been my motivator for becoming a doctor. After so many decades of practice without untutored interference, I finally encountered inane regulations and bureaucratic directives for the first time. Bureaucrats took my arguments in defence of my patients and in defiance of medical bureaucracy to be dangerous (no patient had complained, or suffered any ill-effect of my clinical management). What concerned them most must have been my disrespect for their authority, together with my defiant views of their value to society (see Appendix 2).

Doctors are much more likely to achieve a clinical record like mine using humility rather than arrogance. Like many others, I achieved it simply by being of service, and by having insight enough to manage clinical risk safely, while applying clinical knowledge and experience to the practice of medicine and invasive cardiology. None of this has ever been the remit of a lawyer or medical bureaucrat, yet they have the authority to interfere as the most appropriate people to safeguard the public.

Who should the public trust more? Doctors known to be safe by patients, or medically untrained officials, bureaucrats and regulators?

Those who choose the latter need to provide evidence that both patient morbidity and mortality have benefited from medical bureaucratic intervention. They have made our sacred cow sick. The NHS in the hands of bureaucrats, has become critically ill, and now has a poor prognosis. Novel systemic change is now needed urgently, but unfortunately the suggestions of those who know most about medical practice will fall on deaf ears attached to ignorant, bureaucratically-indoctrinated brains.

I wish all doctors, nurses, and other carers luck when trying to navigate a safe path through the many artificial regulatory pitfalls created by those who justifiably envy the capability medical professionals possess, and will continue to use in the dedicated care of others.

Glossary

Acute: recent onset.

AF: Atrial fibrillation. An irregular heartbeat.

Angiogram: video X-rays of dye being injected into an artery. Helps define blockages.

Atheroma: the build-up of cholesterol and calcified compounds in arteries.

Atherosclerosis: Same as atheroma.

BAME: Black, Asian and Minority Ethnic.

b.d: Medication given twice daily (bi diem).

Benzodiazepine: a class of tranquillizer drugs used for sedation.

Beta-Blocker: drug that slows the heart by blocking the effects of sympathetic drive.

BLOB: BLindingly OBvious.

BNF: British National Formulary.

Bureaucrat. From the French '*bureau*' (desk), and the Greek '*kratos*' (power or rule).

CABG: Coronary Artery Bypass Graft.

CAD: Coronary Artery Disease

Cardiac Infarction: Death of a segment of heart tissue (heart attack).

Cardiovascular Disease: disease of the heart, arteries and veins.

Chronic: Long-term.

Coronary: arteries of the heart.

Coronary bypass: see CABG.

CQC: Care Quality Commission.

CVA: Cerebrovascular accident (a stroke). Due to haemorrhage or clot.

CVS: Cardiovascular System.

Diverticular mass. The large bowel (colon) can have pouches in its wall which get inflamed.

'Dripped and sucked': An intravenous drip together with a stomach tube to suck out contents.

'Drexit': 'Doctor Exit'. Many junior doctors now quitting their jobs.

DVT: Deep Vein Thrombosis.

ESR: Erythrocyte Sedimentation Rate: a blood test index of inflammation.

FRCOG: Fellow of the Royal College of Obstetricians and Gynaecologists.

FRCS: Fellow of the Royal College of Surgeons.

Genome: Our genes, found in every cell. The inherited DNA structure that helps define us.

GMC: General Medical Council.

Hyper: Increased

Hyperglycaemia: Increased blood glucose.

Hypertension: High blood pressure.

Hypo: under. Hypotension = low blood pressure.

Hypovolaemia: Underfilling of the circulation (as in blood loss and dehydration).

IHD: Ischaemic Heart Disease (narrowed arteries with less blood reaching heart muscle).

ITU: Intensive Therapy Unit.

JVP (Jugular Venous Pressure): neck vein pressure as a measure of heart function.

LV: Left ventricle (main heart pumping chamber).

LVH: Left Ventricular Hypertrophy: increased heart muscle with hypertension, etc.

Metastases and metastatic: cancerous tumours that have widely spread.

Morbidity: the occurrence of any medical condition or disease.

MRCP: Member of the Royal College of Physicians

Neoplastic. Cancerous pathology.

NICE: National Institute for Care and Health Excellence.

NSTEMI: No ST Elevation seen in Myocardial Infarction. No ECG changes seen.

OPD: Out Patient Department.

OTC: Over The Counter preparation.

PA: Pulmonary artery.

PE: Pulmonary Embolus (clot that has travelled to the lung).

PSA: Prostate Specific Antigen (blood test for prostate cancer).

PSA: Professional Standards Authority.

Pulmonary embolism: a clot travelling from a leg vein (as an embolus) to lodge in a lung.

RCP: Royal College of Physicians.

Royal Colleges. Those for physicians, surgeons, obstetricians and gynaecologists, and GPs.

Septicaemia: Blood-born infection that can affect all internal organs and cause collapse and death.

Sepsis. The same as septicaemia.

Statins: A class of pharmaceuticals that can lower blood cholesterol.

STEMI: Heart attack with ECG changes (ST Elevation in Myocardial Infarction).

Stents, stenting: Insertion of a metal cage within an artery to stop it narrowing.

Thromboembolism: Clots (thrombus /thrombi) when travelling in blood vessels are called emboli.

URTI: Upper Respiratory Tract Infection (such as tonsillitis and bronchitis)

Bibliography & Notes

The State of UK Medical Practice

Matthew Syed: Is the NHS Broken? (*Dispatches*, 28/10/2021, Channel 4 TV).

The King's Fund (2018). In their document (combined with The Health Foundation and Nuffield Trust) *Budget 2018: What it means for health and social care.* Pages 2 & 3, they state: 'As things stand, the planned costs need to be met from within the current DHSC budget, meaning the increase to the remaining DHSC resource and capital budget combined (total DEL) will be just 2.7% in real terms next year, to £132.7bn.'

Jennifer Dixon, Chief Executive of the Heath Foundation, said that, 'you get what you pay for!' (*Dispatches*, 28/10/2021, Channel 4 TV).

'*Staffing matters; funding counts*'. The Health Foundation. July 2016. www. Health.org.uk

PLAB tests (Professional and Linguistic Assessments Board). GMC: Registration and Licensing. www.gmc-uk.org

Royal College of Surgeons (RCS). *Report: Waiting Times Survey.* 28th January 2020. The report reflects the views of 421 surgeons who worked in NHS hospitals across England in November 2019.

Cancer mortality per million in the UK was recently 216. In Holland this is 206, in France 197, in Germany 192, in Spain 181, and in Sweden 173. These figures do not support the idea that the UK offers 'world beating' cancer management. Source: The Health Foundation.

Prof. Chris Ham, a health policy academic, said, 'Doing more of the same is no longer an option. The NHS will have to do things differently by embracing innovation and becoming much more efficient in how it uses the £130bn it spends each year.'

Manchester University NHS Foundation Trust, and University Hospitals Birmingham receive approximately four negligence claims each week. Sources: Matthew Syed. *Dispatches*, Channel 4 TV, 18/10/2021, and The Health Foundation.

Prof. Alan Merry, Head of the School of Medicine, Auckland, NZ., RSM Conference: 'When Things go Wrong' (26th Oct. 2018).

BMJ Editorial. BMJ (2004) 11; 329 (7466) 583. 'Ethnic Profile of the doctors in the UK'. Of 81,000 UK doctors surveyed in 2004, 63% were from a white ethnic origin, 23% were Asian, 4% black, 1% of mixed race, and 7% other.

In 2011, 29% of those living in Newham identified their ethnic group within the 'White' category. In 2021 this had increased to 30.8% (Office for National Statistics. *Census 2021*).

Wilson, E.O. Oxford Essential Quotations (4th Ed. 2016). 'The real problem of humanity is the following: we have Paleolithic emotions, medieval institutions, and godlike technology.'

The Intergovernmental Panel on Climate Change (IPCC) in August 2021 stated that 'Many of the changes observed in the climate are unprecedented in thousands, if not hundreds of thousands of years . . .' https://www. ipcc.ch.

Film. *The Wizard of Oz*. MGM. 1939.

Bambra, Clare (2016). *Health Divides: Where You Live Can Kill You*. p. 138, Bristol University Press.

Yuval Noah Harari (*Sapiens*, Penguin. Vintage, Random House. 2011, Chapter 8).

George Bernard Shaw (*Pygmalion*. 1913).

Dennis Campbell, in *The Guardian newspaper* (December 2019) 'Out of four million attendances in UK A&E's (between 2016 and 2019), 5449 died while waiting for admission to a hospital bed.'

Yuval Noah Harari. *Homo Deus*. 2015. Random House.

Niccoló Machiavelli, (Book VI of *The Art of War* (1521).

Elton, Caroline (2018): *Also Human: The Inner Lives of Doctors*. Cornerstone.

Storring, Dr. Roderick. *The Tyranny of a System*. *The NHS*. Amazon. (ISBN 10 1521840814)

Iacobucci, Gareth (2021). 'Burnout is harming GPs' health and patient care.'

BMJ 2021;374:n1823 http://dx.doi.org/10.1136/bmj.n1823 Published: 19 July 2021.

Quotes Shan Hussain, a GP in Nottingham. 'We have many measures such as appraisals, revalidation, CQC inspections . . . which have very little scientific evidence to support their use yet are imposed unilaterally upon us and cause remarkable distress.'

US Health Maintenance Organisations (HMOs).

Barker W.F., Hickman E.B., Harper J.A., Lungren J., Barker W.F., et al. (1997). 'Venous interruption for pulmonary embolism: The illustrative case of Richard M. Nixon.' Ann Vasc Surg. 1997 Jul;11(4):387-90. doi: 10.1007/s100169900066. Ann Vasc Surg. 1997. PMID: 9236996.

Mrs. Margaret Thatcher. The Health Foundation, 25 January 1988.

Obakata, Haruko, et al (2014). *Stimulus-triggered fate conversion of somatic cells into pluripotency.* Nature 505 (7485), 641–647; doi:10.1038/nature12968.

Obakata, Haruko. (Japan Times, May 2019). 'When I dream about enjoying the company of people who I'll never see again, it seems unreal. This fills my heart with pain.'

Matthu, Dr. Raj. (2010). Express newspaper, Padraic Flanagan. 'NHS wastes £6m paying top doctor to stay away from work

Francis, Robert (2010). The Francis Inquiry. Report of the Mid

Staffordshire NHS Foundation Trust Public Inquiry: Executive Summary. Google Books (ISBN 9780102964394)

Kapur, Professor Narinder. Dismissed in July 2012 by NHS. *'Top doctor unfairly sacked from Addenbrooke's dedicates lifetime achievement award to 'all sacked NHS whistleblowers.'*

Cambridgeshire Live (31 MAR 2017), by Freya Leng.

'The Weekend Effect'. A NIHR-funded study: 2018doi: 10.3310/signal-000539).

The Control of Medical Practice

Voltaire. (1764). *Dictionnaire Philosophique.*

Rustin, Bayard. And Michael G. Long (2012). *I Must Resist: Bayard Rustin's Life in Letters* . Publisher: City Lights.

Rumpole of the Bailey, 'Rumpole and the Golden Thread'. *(1983)*. Based on John Mortimer's book. Thames Television Ltd.

Huxley, Aldous, (1932). *Brave New World.* Chatto and Windus.

Homer, *The Odyssey.* Penguin Classics. 2003.

Sellu, David. (2019) *Did He Save Lives?*, David Sellu. Sweetcroft Publishing.

Graeber, David (2015). *The Utopia of Rules*, p82. Melville House.

Parkinson, C, Northcote (1958). *Parkinson's Law or the Pursuit of Progress* published by John Murray.

Powell, Dr. Mark, and Gifford, Jonathon (2018). *Machiavellian Intelligence.* LID Publishing.

Plato, *The Republic* (c.375 BC). Socrates asks, 'Are some citizens more valuable than others?'

Siedentop, Larry. (2014). *Inventing the Individual.* London, Allen Lane.

Louis XIV (13/4/1655) *Devant les Parlementaires Parisiens.* Summarily dismissed all of his advisers and bureaucrats, remarking: *'L'état, c'est moi.'*

Junior Doctors Strike (for one day) on the 12th January 2016.

Reagan, Ronald. 'The primary role of government is to protect its citizens. The primary function of the law is to protect individuals from one another. Who is to protect individuals from the government and the law? Where government has gone beyond its limits is in deciding to protect us from ourselves.' Quotes. From BrainyQuote.com

Plato, Socrates: 'Ignorance is the greatest crime.' *The Dialogues of Plato,* Volume 4, (1895) translated by B. Jewett, professor of Greek, University of Oxford. Plato (428-348 BC).

The Bawa Gaba Case. The High Court ruling was over-turned on 13th of August 2018.

Horsfal, Sarndrah. *GMC Internal Review* (2014). 'During the period under review (2005–2013), there were 28 reported cases in the GMC's records where a doctor committed suicide, or where suicide was possible, while under their investigation procedures.'

Dr. Hendrik Beerstecher. Pulse Magazine (August, 2019).

GDPR legislation. The Health and Social Care Act 2008. Article 6, (e).

Good Medical Practice. GMC Publication, 1995.

Shakespeare, William. *Julius Caesar*, act 3, scene 1.

Film *Apocalypse Now* (United Artists, 1979).

Cohen, Josh (2013) *The Private Life*, p39. Granta.

Sowell, Thomas. Source:https://www.brainyquote.com/quotes/thomas_sowell_392884.

Ross, Nick (2021). RSM webinar *'When things go wrong. Doctors in the dock'.*

Future Medical Practice

Reynolds, Alan. 'How to Model Simulated 2.2 Million U.S. Deaths from COVID-19'. Cato Institute, April 21,2020. Cites Professor Ferguson's 'sensational death estimates' of 510000 COVID-19 deaths in the UK. (Imperial College, London)

Box, George, E.P. 'Science and Statistics'. *Journal of American Statistical Association* (1976). Vol 71, 356, p791.

Florence Nightingale, Pamphlet 1858: 'Notes on matters affecting the Health, Efficiency and Hospital Administration of the British Army'.

'*Good Medical Practice*'. GMC Publication, 1995.

Stephenson, Jo: Nursing Times (23/4/2014): '6Cs' nursing values to be rolled out to all NHS staff.'

Haslam, Prof. David. Chair of NICE. (2/10/2015). RCGP Meeting. *'Prevention is better than cure.'*

Harari, Yuval Noah (2011), *Sapiens. A Brief History of Humankind.* Vintage.

Film *Back to the Future* (1985), Universal Pictures.

Pulse. 'Pulse survey reveals GPs working beyond safe limits'. (May 2019). Cogora.

Niven, Dr. James, Medical Officer for Health in Manchester. Report on the Epidemic of Influenza in Manchester, 1918-19.

Hunter, John (1728-1793). Anatomist and surgeon at St. George's, Hyde Park Corner, London. From inscription on a bust at St. George's Hospital, Tooting. London

Snow, C.P. (1959). *Two Cultures, and the Scientific Revolution.* OUP.

Yes, Minister. BBC TV series 1980-82.

Hayek, F. A., (1967), 'The Theory of Complex Phenomena: A Precocious Play on the Epistemology of Complexity'. Originally published in 'Studies in Philosophy and Economics', London, UK: Routledge & Kegan Paul, pp. 22-42.

David Dighton

Epilogue

Maximillian Weber (1864-1920). *The Theory of Social and Economic Organisation*, 1920. Also an essay: On Bureaucracy. See Weber's *Rationalism and Modern Society*, 2015, pp. 73–127, edited and translated by Tony Waters and Dagmar Waters, New York: Palgrave MacMillan.

Appendix 1

Me and the GMC

What follows is the letter I wrote to my solicitor, and conveyed to my barrister and Tribunal members (MPTS at the GMC):

Letter (29/10/19, 8.00am) to solicitor
Alex Leslie, Radcliffes LeBrasseur, London.

Dear Alex,
With much regret, I have decided to resign from the MPTS proceedings, and to resign my licence to practise medicine with immediate effect. I will, therefore, not be attending the Tribunal further.

It is my wish that the reasons for my retiring from proceedings are presented to the MPTS so that they may be duly recorded.

Please give my sincere respects and apologies to Stephen, and thank him for his splendid representation of my case. He was battling against obviously antagonistic panel members, malign GMC desires, and the ineptitude of their advocate.

In my opinion, the Tribunal, as constituted, has insufficient knowledge of the patient; me, as a senior experienced physician, and my particular practice (which largely exists to deal with those patients (like 'Patient A'), who was failed by NHS GPs and hospital services to meet her clinical needs).

It is clear to me from the questions I was asked under oath yesterday, that neither the Tribunal panel members, nor the barrister for the GMC, have any idea of the nature of clinical diagnosis, or of the clinical management of even the simplest of clinical cases; let alone challenging cases like Patient A.

I now find myself at ideological odds with the attitudes and direction of the GMC expressed in the proceedings.

I have concluded that the MPTS process and the GMC corporate body, representing as it does a legally-oriented rather than a medically-oriented body, is unfit to judge my clinical involvement with Patient A.

I have based my opinion on multiple examples of the gross deficiency of understanding of clinical matters, expressed in camera yesterday (28/10/2019 MPTS). I will quote but two examples:

It was regarded yesterday as a deficiency that I offered no apology to Patient A. This makes no sense and illustrates a total lack of understanding of the case by the GMC's barrister. It would be like having to apologise to the burglar I chased from my house: firstly because he was not allowed enough time to steal more of my goods, and secondly because I exposed him to undue risk, having forced him to use a ladder from my bedroom window, rather than use my stairs to escape. Patent nonsense.

Given that patient A apologised to me many times for the

trouble she had caused me, an apology from me would have been entirely inappropriate. I quote this as a symptomatic example of the obvious misunderstanding of the whole case expressed during yesterday's proceedings. There was no sense to my expressing contrition or regret for my actions when I successfully managed her for many years and kept her from harm. The truth is that neither the patient nor I ever had any faith in the NHS to handle her case safely and appropriately. Being an addict, she was always at risk, but her risk of harm would in my judgement have been far greater in the hands of NHS providers (her opinion also as an ex-NHS nurse, and that of her husband, as well as (I contend), that of most of my 20,000 private patients!).

Second, to be asked by a GP panel member to explain how I knew when cases were 'simple and straightforward' (like a grazed knee, or a common cold), rather than complicated like sepsis, is a question for a GP trainee, not an experienced hospital physician like me. My role has always been to handle sick, 'complicated' cases, as well as the diagnostic and clinical managerial incompetence of many NHS GPs.

I quote these two as examples of the obvious unfitness of the Tribunal panel to grasp (1) the true nature of Patient A (a deceitful drug addict, but one with whom I had an effective and successful doctor patient relationship), and (2) of me, and (3) my practice and its distinguishing attributes in relation to NHS providers. For these reasons, I have no faith in the reliability of the forthcoming judgement of the MPTS panel, whatever it may be.

The unfitness of both the GMC and CQC as corporate, legally constituted bodies, judging doctors is another matter of concern to me. I have addressed this in a book to be published later.

The corporate attempts of the GMC and CQC to standardise the actions of doctors (partly through using 'guidelines' as 'fixed rules'), and to regard all patients having standardised clinical needs, is unrepresentative (and, therefore, unscientific), impracticable, and untenable: something I strongly disagree with. It will lead to harm and I can support it no longer.

I am fully aware that I will be among very many others (doctors and nurses) who have already resigned the medical profession for allied reasons; all of which relate back to the attempts of medical bureaucracy to corporatise medicine.

I guess the enquiries into my notes will continue, and the Tribunal's judgement and ruling will have procedural consequences. I will, therefore, undoubtedly be in need of your further advice on how best to finalise my career.

I have been so impressed by the expertise and advice you have shown me personally. Having experts like you, Roger, Stephen, and your respective team members on my side means that I have had the very best of legal representation. I will remain thankful to you all.

Yours sincerely,

David Dighton

What followed one year later was that the Public Services Authority became involved once they realised the GMC were happy to let me retire. As a legal precedent which you can read about in the BMJ, they applied to the High Court to force a decision on the GMC - to strike me off the Medical Register. They wanted me never to return as a doctor again (aged seventy-seven years at the time). Remember that I had never harmed a patient, or been complained about. Perhaps my greatest crime was to show contempt for those who regulate the medical profession.

Following that, the CQC categorised me as unfit to be a registered provider and manager of Loughton Clinic. Corporations can anonymously do what they choose. The problem is that they can remain anonymous and detached from humanity, and carry on regardless. I would argue that the harm done by removing one effective medical practitioner (with the capacity to save lives, and remove pain and morbidity) is more than any contribution made a bureaucrat.

The directive 'terminate with extreme prejudice' first arose in the Vietnam war. The character Jerry (played by Jerry Ziesmer), in the film *Apocalypse Now* (United Artists, 1979), used these words.

The phrase would seem to typify the intent of the PSA in my case. So heinous were my prescribing crimes that the Public Services Authority (PSA) challenged the decisions of the MPTS and GMC. They directed I should be 'struck off', rather than have voluntary erasure (as agreed by the GMC). They wanted to stop any chance of my returning to work as a certified doctor, even though I retired one year before, at age seventy-six. The High Court upheld their desire. Their ruling was later ratified by the GMC in November 2020. My advisers predicted I couldn't win, so I had no inclination to waste my time further.

For the PSA this was an Irenic victory (one where the loser loses very little), rather than a Pyrrhic one where the victor pays a heavy price for a little gain. In my case the victor paid with public money (partly mine), not their own. They had nothing to lose, something common to many faceless organisations. Those who work for them are free to exert their power without personal consequence.

This will continue while the NHS, and all who work in

its controlling bureaucratic pyramid, regard themselves as more important than doctors, nurses, and patients. While this continues, medical bureaucracy in the UK will never be fit for purpose.

In my case they failed to appreciate that my private practice was atypical (cases seen in general medicine, cardiology, with some general practice, with plenty of time afforded to each patient), and substantially different from that of any NHS doctor, including the Birmingham NHS GP member on my particular MPTS Tribunal. My practice differed greatly from NHS GP practices. The time I always made available for my patients was considerably more; the depth of personal knowledge I had of each patient was much more extensive (lengthy consultation times being the *sine qua non* for this); there was greater availability (patients could contact me easily, and in person), and unchanging continuity. All these were substantial differences, but they considered none of them (my barrister informed me they would regard them as hearsay and irrelevant). These differences are, however, key to patient safety, and define the quality of a medical service. It is why patients paid to consult me for forty-five years, despite competition from the 'free' NHS service available to them.

In ignorance of all these crucial differences, they judged me as if I was an NHS GP (the only practice the members of the Tribunal could relate to). Their judgement of me as 'unsafe' might have applied to an NHS GP practice, but not mine. My past record meant nothing, I was told. That they ignored the fact that no patient of mine (including the three whose medication they reviewed) came to any harm in forty-six years suggested they were unwilling to consider how life is at the coalface. Do they really believe that a healthy pilot who has flown daily for fifty-three years and never crashed will not be safe to fly tomorrow? In believing that a risk-free world should exist, they must punish doctors to exclude the possibility of their being wrong, hardly the application of wisdom as a member of the public might understand it. Their overriding need is for failsafe judgements and punishments.

Because the MPTS and I were singing from different song sheets, the time came to resign from the proceedings, resign from medical practice, and move on.

Appendix 2

Please note: Apart from headings, my comments are those in bold letters.

Authority appeal upheld in case of GMC and Dr Dighton
04 Dec 2020

Background to the appeal

Dr David Dighton specialised in cardiology but also had a private practice as a General Practitioner (GP) (**general physician, actually**). He had no formal training as a GP (**I was once a principal GP partner**). Patient A became one of his general practice patients in 2011 and he prescribed a large number of drugs to her for around six years (**over which period she came to no harm. Luck, obviously!**). These included strong painkillers, sleeping tablets, antidepressants and tranquilisers. Over the same period the patient had also been prescribed several of the same drugs from her own GP. Dr Dighton had not notified Patient A's GP that he was treating her as a private patient and prescribing drugs (**Incorrect. But the GP I informed retired during the six years I treated her**). In 2017, the patient was diagnosed with prescription drug dependency (amongst other things). Dr Dighton's actions took place against a background of interventions by the GMC:

1. In 2011 he was issued with a letter of advice from the GMC relating to his prescribing, and
2. In 2016 he appeared before and received a warning from the Investigation Committee in a case relating to his prescribing of benzodiazepines (**they forgot to mention that I withdrew all my patients from these drugs under the supervision of a GP**).

The case brought against Dr Dighton by the GMC

The case that was brought by the GMC to the Medical Practitioners Tribunal (Tribunal) alleged that the doctor had:

- Prescribed excessively a number of different drugs to Patient A;
- Failed adequately to assess (**they doubted my clinical acumen**) or appropriately refer her to mental health services (**private doctors cannot refer directly to NHS**

psychiatrists, and she refused anyway).

- Kept inadequate records (**this is true. I saw her two to three times every week and the notes would have been ditto, ditto, etc.**).
- Failed to inform her GP that he had issued the patient with prescriptions (**incorrect**);
- Lacked adequate expertise to treat her (**so they say, based on a lack of certification. Not quite the same thing!**).

In reaching its conclusion on impairment the Tribunal expressed

> *'grave concerns in relation to Dr Dighton's poor practice over a six-year period despite an advice letter in 2011 and a warning in 2016'. It described 'his lack of insight' as 'intractable'* (**my attitude to the expertise of bureaucrats was intractable**) *such that 'he is unlikely to remediate and there is a material risk of repetition.'* (**correct**). *The combination of lack of insight* (**having read this book would you say I had any insight worth having?**), *unfocused training* (**so experience means nothing?**), *lack of any apology* (**the patient was entirely happy with me and no apology was appropriate**) *and lack of reflective practice* (**how much more reflection time is necessary when one sees the patient 3 times every week for six years?**) *meant that the risk of repetition could not be regarded as low.'*

Before the Tribunal made the decision on the appropriate sanction, the doctor gave evidence. He stated he had stopped working as a GP following a discussion with an adviser from the CQC who had impressed on him that GP work was a speciality (**not true**); he referred to his clinical experience from the 1970s of prescribed drugs and that he had been deceived by the patient who he described as 'clever and manipulative' (**clever enough to dupe me**). By prescribing drugs in a manner that was different to established practice, he was '*trying to make an academic point.*' (**They have not understood me. Why should lawyers understand anything about medical management, some reasons for which might be academic? I have always advocated off-piste prescribing as an academic exercise when all other doctors have failed to help a patient**). He had not apologised to the patient, saying that she was happy with her treatment. He rejected the suggestion that he posed a risk to patients in the future (**were my 20,000 patients seen over forty-five years wrong about the risk I presented?**); he had removed '*all contentious issues.*' The Tribunal's decision was to suspend Dr Dighton for twelve months with review.

Why did we appeal?

We decided to appeal this decision on the basis that the suspension order was insufficient to protect the public and that the registrant ought to have been struck off (**lawyers making medical risk assessments**). We argued that the Tribunal's approach to deciding the sanction was irrational and wrong (**a specious claim. The word 'irrational' means 'not logical or reasonable'. Clearly the wrong word**); the Tribunal had failed to take sufficient regard of the relevant guidance on sanctions and finally that the Tribunal took an irrational (**that**

inappropriate word again) approach to the registrant's insight into his misconduct (**this is an illogical conclusion. Her only point is that she does not think the MPTS followed the sanction guidelines**).

A few weeks after we lodged our appeal, the doctor applied for and was granted voluntary erasure from the GMC register. A few days later the GMC notified the parties that this decision would be stayed pending the outcome of our appeal.

At the hearing we argued that a suspension order and a voluntary erasure order would be insufficient for the protection of the public. This was a particularly serious case (**where nobody came to harm, just as no patient was ever harmed in forty-five years of my private practice**) where the correct outcome was erasure and any other outcome would undermine the importance of upholding confidence in the medical profession (**an existential matter which they cannot judge**) and the importance of maintaining standards (**while treating patients as human rather than numbers, perhaps?**).

Our submissions on seriousness referred to the actions of the doctor in prescribing addictive medicines to a vulnerable patient (**clever, but not vulnerable**) whom he considered to demonstrate addictive behaviour. The doctor (who did not attend the appeal hearing) (**I had already retired**) repeated his submissions that this appeal and the hearing were unnecessary given the decision of the GMC to grant his application for voluntary erasure.

Outcome

The Court allowed the appeal, quashed the suspension order and substituted its own order for erasure. The judgment includes mention of:

- The fact that the Authority's appeal was properly brought before the Court and that our appeal right could be frustrated if a registrant was able to avoid the scrutiny of an appeal by opting for voluntary erasure.
- A reminder to panels that they are bound to apply the sanctions guidance properly and they are under a duty to reach a decision on sanction in a way that would protect the public.
- In relation to assessments of insight and the prospect of developing insight, the Court pointed to the fact that the Tribunal had found the registrant had no insight into his misconduct, blamed his patient (**both wrong**), and had not apologised: therefore the MPT's decision to suspend (and in effect give the doctor another chance to develop insight) was unreasonable and inconsistent with the evidence before it. In a previous NMC appeal brought by the PSA the Court had referred to this as '*an exercise in wishful thinking that the panel had engaged in*'.
- The Court also stated that statutory regulation of the medical profession is designed to prevent the sort of risks which the doctor had caused his patient and his '*resistance to regulatory control*' was relevant to his lack of insight and means that he cannot be trusted to practise as a doctor again. (**Here we have the real reason**

for their discontent – my 'resistance to regulatory control'. They got that right at least!

Index

www.ingramcontent.com/pod-product-compliance
Lightning Source LLC
Chambersburg PA
CBHW051714020426
42333CB00014B/984